Laboratory Manual and Workbook in
MICROBIOLOGY

APPLICATIONS TO PATIENT CARE

FIFTH EDITION

Laboratory Manual and Workbook in MICROBIOLOGY

APPLICATIONS TO PATIENT CARE

JOSEPHINE A. MORELLO, A.M., PH.D.
Director of Clinical Microbiology Laboratories, Professor, Departments of Pathology and Medicine,
The University of Chicago, Illinois

HELEN ECKEL MIZER, R.N., A.B., M.S., M.ED.
Formerly Professor, Department of Nursing,
Western Connecticut State University, Danbury, Connecticut

MARION E. WILSON, M.A., PH.D., D.L. (HON.)
Formerly Director of Microbiology,
Public Health Laboratory Services, New York City Department of Health

WCB **Wm. C. Brown Publishers**
Dubuque, Iowa • Melbourn, Australia • Oxford, England

Book Team

Editor *Megan Johnson*
Developmental Editor *Jane DeShaw*
Production Editor *Cathy Ford Smith*
Designer *Christopher E. Reese*
Art Editor *Jodi Wagner*
Photo Editor *Carrie Burger*
Permissions Coordinator *Mavis M. Oeth*

Wm. C. Brown Publishers
A Division of Wm. C. Brown Communications, Inc.

Vice President and General Manager *Beverly Kolz*
Vice President, Director of Sales and Marketing *Virginia S. Moffat*
Marketing Manager *Christopher T. Johnson*
Advertising Manager *Janelle Keeffer*
Director of Production *Colleen A. Yonda*
Publishing Services Manager *Karen J. Slaght*

Wm. C. Brown Communications, Inc.

President and Chief Executive Officer *G. Franklin Lewis*
Corporate Vice President, President of WCB Manufacturing *Roger Meyer*
Vice President and Chief Financial Officer *Robert Chesterman*

Cover © Tom Grill/Comstock

Earlier editions by Marion E. Wilson, Martin H. Weisburd, and Helen
Eckel Mizer. Copyright © 1974 by Macmillan Publishing Co., Inc., by
Marion E. Wilson, Martin H. Weisburd, Helen Eckel Mizer, and
Josephine A. Morello. Copyright © 1979 by Macmillan Publishing Co.,
Inc., by Josephine A. Morello, Helen Eckel Mizer, and Marion E.
Wilson, copyright © 1984 by Macmillan Publishing Co., Inc.

A Times Mirror Company

ISBN 0-697-13784-8

Some of the laboratory experiments included in this text may be
hazardous if materials are handled improperly or if procedures are
conducted incorrectly. Safety precautions are necessary when you are
working with chemicals, glass test tubes, hot water baths, sharp
instruments, and the like, or for any procedures that generally require
caution. Your school may have set regulations regarding safety
procedures that your instructor will explain to you. Should you have
any problems with materials or procedures, please ask your instructor
for help.

Printed in the United States of America by Wm. C. Brown Communications, Inc.,
2460 Kerper Boulevard, Dubuque, IA 52001

10   9   8   7   6   5   4   3   2   1

CONTENTS

Preface   *vii*

PART 1
Basic Techniques of Microbiology   *1*

Section I.   **Orientation to the Microbiology Laboratory**   *3*

Warning   *3*
Safety Procedures and Precautions   *3*
General Laboratory Directions   *4*

Exercise
1. The Microscope   *7*
2. Handling and Examining Cultures   *15*

Section II.   **Microscopic Morphology of Microorganisms**   *23*

Exercise
3. Hanging-Drop and Wet-Mount Preparations   *25*
4. Simple Stains   *31*

Section III.   **Differential Stains**   *35*

Exercise
5. Gram Stain   *37*
6. Acid-Fast Stain   *41*
7. Special Stains   *45*

Section IV.   **Cultivation of Microorganisms**   *51*

Exercise
8. Culture Media   *53*
9. Pure Culture Technique   *57*
10. Pour-Plate and Subculture Techniques   *63*
11. Culturing Microorganisms from the Environment   *69*

PART 2
Destruction of Microorganisms   *73*

Section V.   **Physical Antimicrobial Agents**   *75*

Exercise
12. Moist and Dry Heat   *77*
13. The Autoclave   *81*

Section VI.   **Chemical Antimicrobial Agents**   *89*

Exercise
14. Disinfectants   *91*
15. Antimicrobial Agents (Antimicrobial Susceptibility Testing)   *95*

PART 3
Diagnostic Microbiology in Action   *103*

General Considerations   *103*
Microbiology at the Bedside   *103*
Precautions for Handling Specimens or Cultures   *104*
Normal Flora of the Body   *105*

Section VII.   **Principles of Diagnostic Microbiology: Culture of Clinical Specimens; Identifying Isolated Microorganisms**   *107*

Exercise
16. Primary Media for Isolation of Microorganisms   *109*
17. Some Metabolic Activities of Bacteria   *115*
18. Activities of Bacterial Enzymes   *121*

Section VIII. **Microbiology of the Respiratory Tract** *127*

Exercise

19. Streptococci, Pneumococci, and Enterococci *129*
20. Staphylococci *147*
21. *Klebsiella* and *Haemophilus* *153*
22. Corynebacteria and *Bordetella* *159*
23. Clinical Specimens from the Respiratory Tract *165*

Section IX. **Microbiology of the Intestinal Tract** *173*

Exercise

24. The *Enterobacteriaceae* (Enteric Bacilli) *175*
25. Clinical Specimens from the Intestinal Tract *189*

Section X. **Microbiology of the Urinary and Genital Tracts** *195*

Exercise

26. Urine Culture Techniques *197*
27. *Neisseria* and Spirochetes *203*

Section XI. **Microbial Pathogens Requiring Special Laboratory Techniques** *211*

Exercise

28. Anaerobic Bacteria *213*
29. Mycobacteria *221*
30. Mycoplasmas, Rickettsiae, Chlamydiae, and Viruses *225*
31. Fungi: Yeasts and Molds *231*
32. Protozoa and Animal Parasites *239*

PART 4

Serological Procedures *247*

Exercise

33. Serological Identification of Microorganisms *249*
34. Serological Identification of Patients' Antibodies *253*

PART 5

Applied (Sanitary) Microbiology *257*

Exercise

35. Bacteriologic Analysis of Water *259*
36. Bacteriologic Analysis of Milk *263*

APPENDICES

I. Notes to Instructors *269*
II. Preparation of Reagents *277*
III. Preparation and Storage of Media *279*
IV. Sources and Maintenance of Stock Cultures *281*
V. Audiovisual (AV) and Source Material *285*

PREFACE

This laboratory manual and workbook, now in its fifth edition, maintains its original emphasis on the basic principles of diagnostic microbiology for students preparing to enter the allied health professions. It remains oriented primarily toward meeting the interests and needs of those who will be directly involved in patient care and who wish to learn how microbiological principles should be applied in the practice of their professions. These include nursing students, dental hygienists, dietitians, hospital sanitarians, inhalation therapists, operating room or cardiopulmonary technicians, optometric technicians, physical therapists, and physicians' assistants. For such students, the clinical and epidemiological applications of microbiology often seem more relevant than its technical details. Thus, the challenge for authors of textbooks and laboratory manuals, and for instructors, is to project microbiology into the clinical setting and relate its principles to patient care.

The authors of this manual have emphasized the purposes and functions of the clinical microbiology laboratory in the diagnosis of infectious diseases. The exercises illustrate as simply as possible the nature of laboratory procedures used for isolation and identification of infectious agents, as well as the principles of asepsis, disinfection, and sterilization. The role of the health professional is projected through repeated stress on the importance of the clinical specimen submitted to the laboratory—its proper selection, timing, collection, and handling. Equal attention is given to the applications of aseptic and disinfectant techniques as they relate to practical situations in the care of patients. The manual seeks to provide practical insight and experience rather than to detail the microbial physiology a professional microbiologist must learn. We have approached this revision with a view toward updating basic procedures and reference sources. Every exercise has been carefully reviewed and revised, if necessary, to conform to changing practices in clinical laboratories.

The material is organized into five parts of increasing complexity designed to give students first a sense of familiarity with the nature of microorganisms, then practice in aseptic cultural methods in clinical settings. Part 1 introduces basic techniques of microbiology. It includes general laboratory directions, precautions for handling microorganisms, the use of the microscope, microscopic morphology of microorganisms in wet and stained preparations, pure culture techniques, and an exercise in environmental microbiology. In response to requests from users of this manual, an experiment on the endospore stain has been added.

Part 2 provides instruction and some experience in methods for the destruction of microorganisms, so that students may understand the principles of disinfection and sterilization before proceeding to the study of pathogenic microorganisms. There is an exercise on antimicrobial agents that includes antimicrobial susceptibility testing using the National Committee for Clinical Laboratory Standards (NCCLS) technique, with the latest category designations and inhibition zone interpretations, as well as experiments to determine minimal inhibitory concentrations by the broth dilution method, and bacterial resistance to antimicrobial agents.

The principles learned are then applied to diagnostic microbiology in Part 3. Techniques for collecting clinical specimens (Microbiology at the Bedside) and precautions for handling them are reviewed. A discussion of the Centers for Disease Control and Prevention "universal precautions" for avoiding transmission of bloodborne pathogens is included. The normal flora of various parts of the body is discussed. The five sections of this part cover the principles of diagnostic bacteriology; the microbiology of the respiratory, intestinal, urinary, and genital tracts; and the special techniques required for the recognition of anaerobes, mycobacteria, mycoplasmas, rickettsiae, chlamydiae, viruses, fungi, protozoa, and animal parasites. Sections VIII and IX, dealing respectively with the microbiology of the respiratory and intestinal tracts, present exercises on the common pathogens and normal flora of these areas, followed by exercises dealing with methods for culturing appropriate clinical specimens. Experiments for performing antimicrobial susceptibility tests on relevant isolates from such specimens are also included. In the exercise on streptococci, pneumococci, and enterococci (Section VIII), and other exercises when appropriate, the antigen detection methods for identifying bacteria are included.

Part 4 reviews the principles of serological procedures for identifying microorganisms, including slide agglutination and fluorescent antibody methods, and detection of serum antibodies. Part 5 presents some simple microbiological methods for examining water and milk.

The sequence of the exercises throughout the manual, but particularly in Part 3, is intended to reflect the approach of the diagnostic laboratory to clinical specimens. In each exercise, the student is led to relate the practical world of patient care and clinical diagnosis to the operation of the microbiology laboratory. To learn the normal flora of the body and to appreciate the problem of recognizing clinically significant organisms in a specimen containing mixed flora, students collect and culture their own specimens. Simulated clinical specimens are also used to teach the microbiology of infection. The concept of transmissible infectious disease becomes a reality, rather than a theory, for the student who can see the myriad of microorganisms present on hands, clothes, hair, or environmental objects, and in throat, feces, and urine. Similarly, in learning how antimicrobial susceptibility testing is done, the student acquires insight into the basis for specific drug therapy of infection and the importance of accurate laboratory information.

In acquiring aseptic laboratory technique and a knowledge of the principles of disinfection and sterilization, the student is better prepared for subsequent encounters with pathogenic, transmissible microorganisms in professional practice. The authors believe that one of the most valuable contributions a microbiology laboratory course can make to patient care is to give the student repeated opportunities to understand and develop aseptic techniques through the handling of cultures. Mere demonstrations have little value in this respect. Although the use of pathogenic microorganisms is largely avoided in these exercises, the students are taught to handle all specimens and cultures with respect, since any microorganism may have potential pathogenicity. To illustrate the nature of infectious microorganisms, material to be handled by students includes related "nonpathogenic" species of similar morphological and cultural appearance, and demonstration material presents pathogenic species. Occasional exceptions are made in the case of organisms such as pneumococci, staphylococci, or clostridia that are often encountered, in any case, in the flora of specimens from healthy persons. If the instructor so desires, however, substitutions can be made for these as well.

Teaching flexibility has been sought throughout the manual. There are 36 exercises, many of which contain several experiments. These may be tailored to meet the needs of any prescribed course period, the weekly laboratory hours available, or the interests and capabilities of individual students. The order and emphasis of the material were planned so that the manual could be used in conjunction with the textbook entitled *Microbiology in Patient Care* (Morello, Mizer, Wilson, and Granato, 5th ed., Wm. C. Brown Publishers, Dubuque, Iowa, 1994). Chapters in the text have been cross-referenced at the beginning of each exercise in this manual. However, the manual can be adapted to follow any textbook on basic microbiology appropriate for students entering the allied health field. For the instructor's use, a more complete listing of current literature and other source material is provided in Appendix V.

Each exercise begins with a discussion of the material to be covered, the rationale of methods to be used, and a review of the nature of microorganisms to be studied. In Part 3, tables are frequently inserted to summarize laboratory and/or clinical information concerning the major groups of pathogenic microorganisms. The revised questions that follow each exercise are designed to test the ability of students to relate laboratory information to patient-care situations and to stimulate them to read more widely on each subject presented.

Five appendixes are included to provide instructors with information and assistance in presenting the laboratory course. Appendix I contains a series of notes for instructors. These provide suggestions on how to obtain and prepare the material required for many of the exercises and have been revised to suit the needs of this edition. Appendix II gives methods for preparing the stains and chemical reagents needed for all exercises. Appendix III contains information on the preparation and storage of culture media and lists current sources of media and laboratory supplies. Sources from which reliable stock cultures can be obtained are listed in Appendix IV, and details of practical methods for maintaining stocks are provided. A complete list of all bacterial strains needed for the entire group of exercises can be found in this appendix. Finally, Appendix V lists sources of audiovisual materials, titles and sources of a large number of pertinent films, sources of projection and/or microscope slides for demonstrations, and reference literature on medical microbiology, including several method manuals on diagnostic microbiology. All lists have been revised and updated.

We are grateful to all those professional colleagues who gave generously of their time and expertise to make constructive suggestions regarding the revision of this manual. We owe special thanks to Ms. Paula Chipman (Western Connecticut State University) for her continuing assistance, to Dr. Edward Bottone, Mount Sinai Hospital, New York, for providing us with many of the photographs in the colorplates, and to Mr. Gordon Bowie of the University of Chicago and Mr. Bill Quinnell of Western Connecticut State University for their photographic assistance.

Finally, we acknowledge the role of Wm. C. Brown Publishers in publication of this work. Their many courtesies, extended through Megan Johnson, Associate Acquisitions Editor, and Jane E. DeShaw, Developmental Editor, have encouraged and guided this new edition, and they have been primarily responsible for its production. We are also grateful to Roberta Pettriess of Wichita State University for her helpful review of this manual. For their skillful efforts and expert assistance during the production process, we thank Cathy A. Smith, Production Editor; Chris Reese, Designer; Jodi Wagner, Art Editor; Carrie Burger, Photo Editor; and Mavis Oeth, Permissions Editor.

J. A. M.
H. E. M.
M. E. W.

ONE

Basic Techniques of Microbiology

In beginning the study of medical microbiology, you must learn the basic laboratory techniques used to see microorganisms and to grow them in culture. With knowledge of the microscope and staining techniques, you can study their morphology (features and structures). With an understanding of culture media and how they are used, you can cultivate and study the behavior of these minute organisms that are so important to us in health and disease.

SECTION I

Orientation to the Microbiology Laboratory

Warning

Some of the laboratory experiments included in this text may be hazardous if materials are handled improperly or if procedures are conducted incorrectly. Safety precautions are necessary when you are working with chemicals, glass test tubes, hot water baths, sharp instruments, and the like, or for any procedures that generally require caution. Your school may have set regulations regarding safety procedures that your instructor will explain to you. Should you have any problems with materials or procedures, please ask your instructor for help.

Safety Procedures and Precautions

The microbiology laboratory, whether a classroom or a working diagnostic laboratory, is a place for handling and examining cultures of microorganisms. This type of work must be conducted with good aseptic technique in a scrupulously clean, well-ordered environment. Even if the microorganisms being studied are not considered pathogenic, *any* culture of *any* organism should be handled with respect for its potential pathogenicity.

Each student must quickly learn and continuously practice aseptic laboratory technique. It is important to avoid any risk of contaminating yourself (hands, hair, clothing) or your neighbors with culture material. Also, you must not contaminate the work itself with microorganisms from the environment. The importance of asepsis and proper disinfection is stressed throughout this manual and demonstrated by experiment. Once learned in the laboratory, these techniques apply to virtually every phase of patient care, especially to the collection and handling of specimens ordered for laboratory diagnosis of infectious disease. Such specimens should be handled as meticulously as cultures for the same reasons, so that they do not become sources of infection to others. Sick people are often susceptible to infection by microorganisms that are easily transmitted, especially by contaminated hands. Well-trained professionals caring for the sick should never be responsible for transmitting infection between patients.

In general, all safety procedures and precautions followed in the microbiology laboratory are designed to:

1. *Restrict microorganisms present in specimens or cultures* to the containers in which they are collected, grown, or studied.
2. *Prevent environmental microorganisms* (normally present on hands, hair, clothing, laboratory benches, or in the air) from entering specimens or cultures and interfering with results of studies.

Hands and bench tops are kept clean with disinfectants, protective clothing is worn, hair is controlled, working areas are kept clear of all extraneous items, glass- or plasticware used for specimen collection or culture material is presterilized and capped to prevent entry by unsterile air, and sterile tools are used for transferring specimens or cultures. *Nothing* is placed in the mouth.

Personal conduct in a microbiology laboratory should always be quiet and orderly. The instructor should be consulted promptly whenever problems concerning safety arise. Any student with a fresh, unhealed cut, scratch, burn, or other injury on either hand should report this to the instructor before beginning or continuing the laboratory work of the day. *Thoughtful attention to the principles of safety is required throughout any laboratory course in microbiology.*

General Laboratory Directions

1. Always read the assigned laboratory material *before* the start of the laboratory period.
2. Before entering the laboratory, remove coats, jackets, and other outerwear. These should be left outside the laboratory, together with any books, papers, or other items not needed for the work.
3. To be admitted to the laboratory, each student should wear a fresh, clean, knee-length laboratory coat.
4. At the start and end of each laboratory session, students should clean their assigned bench-top area with a disinfectant solution provided. That space should then be kept neat, clean, and uncluttered throughout each laboratory period.

5. Learn good personal habits from the beginning:

Tie back long hair neatly, away from the shoulders.

Do not wear jewelry to laboratory sessions.

Keep fingers, pencils, and such objects out of your mouth.

Do not smoke, eat, or drink in the laboratory.

Do not lick labels with your tongue (use tap water).

Do not wander about the laboratory (uncontrolled activity can provoke accidents, distract others, and promote contamination).

6. Each student will need matches, bibulous paper, lens paper, a china-marking pencil, and a 100-mm ruler (purchased or provided). A black, waterproof marking pen may be used to mark petri plates and tubes.

7. Keep a complete record of all your experiments, and answer all questions at the end of each exercise. Your completed work can be removed from the manual and submitted to the instructor for evaluation.

8. Discard all cultures and used glassware into the container labeled *CONTAMI-NATED.* (This container will later be sterilized.) Plastic or other disposable items should be discarded separately from glassware in containers to be sterilized.

Never place contaminated pipettes on the bench top.

Never discard contaminated cultures, glassware, pipettes, tubes, or slides in the wastepaper basket or garbage can.

Never discard contaminated liquids or liquid cultures in the sink.

9. If you are in doubt as to the correct procedure, double-check the manual. If doubt continues, consult your instructor. Avoid asking your neighbor for procedural help.

10. If you should spill or drop a culture, *call the instructor immediately* (do this should any type of accident occur).

11. Report any injury to your instructor concerning your hands (before you begin the laboratory work or during the session, depending on when it happened).

12. Students are not permitted to remove specimens, cultures, or equipment from the laboratory, under any circumstances.

13. Before leaving the laboratory, carefully wash and disinfect your hands. Arrange to launder your lab coat so that it will be fresh for the next session.

EXERCISE 1 The Microscope

Reference: Morello, Mizer, Wilson, and Granato, Microbiology in Patient Care, *5th edition, 1994. Chapters 1, 4.*

A good microscope is an essential tool for any microbiology laboratory. There are many kinds of microscopes, but the type most useful in diagnostic work is the *compound microscope.* By means of a series of lenses and a source of bright light, it magnifies and illuminates minute objects such as bacteria and other microorganisms that would otherwise be invisible to the eye. This type of microscope will be used throughout your laboratory course. As you gain experience using it, you will realize how precise it is and how valuable for studying microorganisms present in clinical specimens and in cultures. Even though you may not need to use a microscope in your planned profession, a firsthand knowledge of how to use it can stand you in good stead. In addition, your laboratory experience with it will give you a lasting concept of the existence of living forms too small to be seen with normal vision. Armed with such a view of "invisible" microorganisms, you should be better able to understand their role in transmission of infection.

Purpose	To study the compound microscope and learn A. Its important parts and their functions B. How to focus and use it to study microorganisms C. Its proper care and handling
Materials	An assigned microscope Lens paper Immersion oil A methylene-blue-stained smear of *Candida albicans,* a yeast of medical importance (the fixed, stained smear will be provided by the instructor)

Instructions

A. Important Parts of the Compound Microscope and Their Functions

1. Look at the microscope assigned to you and compare it with the photograph in figure 1.1. Notice that its working parts are set into a sturdy frame consisting of a *base* for support and an *arm* for carrying it. (Note: when lifting and carrying the microscope, always use *both hands;* one to grasp the arm firmly, the other to support the base [fig. 1.2]. *Never* lift it by the part that holds the lenses.)

2. Observe that a flat platform, or *stage* as it is called, extends between the upper lens system and the lower set of devices for providing light. The stage has a hole in the center that permits light from below to pass upward into the lenses above. The object to be viewed is positioned on the stage over this opening so that it is brightly illuminated from below (do not attempt to place your slide on the stage as yet).

   On some microscopes, the stage has clips for holding a glass slide in place, and the slide must be moved by hand when different areas are being examined. Other microscopes have a *mechanical stage* equipped with adjustment knobs for moving the slide in vertical or horizontal directions.

3. The light source is at the base. Most microscopes have a built-in illuminator, as shown in figure 1.1. Others have a mirror attached to the base. The mirror is double-faced, one surface being flat, the other concave. The mirror is used to direct light upward from a lamp placed in front of it, or from a window providing bright daylight. The concave surface is used for daylight to gather scattered, reflected rays of sunlight. The flat surface is used when an electric lamp is the light source.

Figure 1.1 The compound microscope and its parts. Courtesy of Leica Inc., Optical Products Division.

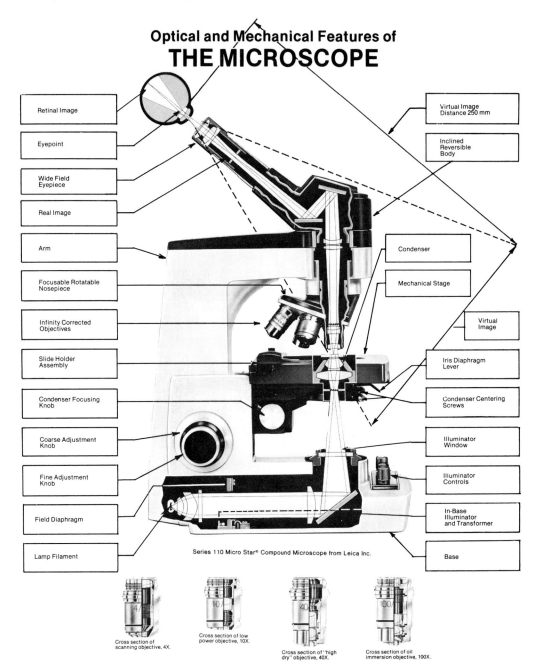

Optical and Mechanical Features of
THE MICROSCOPE

Retinal Image

Eyepoint

Wide Field Eyepiece

Real Image

Arm

Focusable Rotatable Nosepiece

Infinity Corrected Objectives

Slide Holder Assembly

Condenser Focusing Knob

Coarse Adjustment Knob

Fine Adjustment Knob

Field Diaphragm

Lamp Filament

Virtual Image Distance 250 mm

Inclined Reversible Body

Condenser

Mechanical Stage

Virtual Image

Iris Diaphragm Lever

Condenser Centering Screws

Illuminator Window

Illuminator Controls

In-Base Illuminator and Transformer

Base

Series 110 Micro Star® Compound Microscope from Leica Inc.

Cross section of scanning objective, 4X.

Cross section of low power objective, 10X.

Cross section of "high dry" objective, 40X.

Cross section of oil immersion objective, 100X.

4. Light from the mirror or built-in bulb is directed upward through the Abbe *condenser,* placed under the central opening in the stage. The condenser contains lenses that collect and concentrate the light, directing it upward through any object on the stage. It also has a shutter, or *iris diaphragm,* which can be used to adjust the amount of light admitted. A lever (sometimes a rotating knob) is provided on the condenser for operating the diaphragm.

The condenser can be lowered or raised by an adjustment knob. Lowering the condenser decreases the amount of light that reaches the object. This is usually a disadvantage in microbiological work. It is best to keep the condenser fully raised and to adjust light intensity with the iris diaphragm.

Basic Techniques of Microbiology

Figure 1.2 Proper handling of a microscope. Both hands are used when carrying this delicate instrument. Photo by Bill Quinnell, Western Connecticut State University.

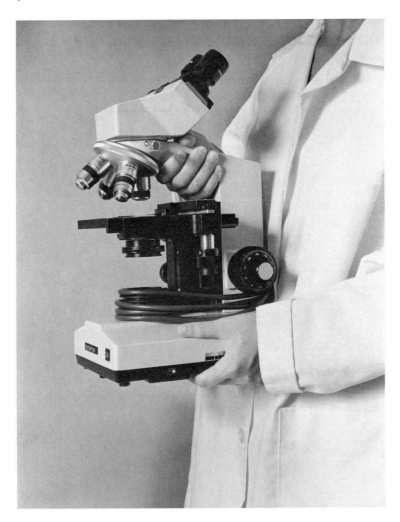

5. Above the stage, attached to the *arm,* a tube holds the magnifying lenses through which the object is viewed. The lower end of the tube is fitted with a *rotating nosepiece* holding three or four *objective lenses.* As the nosepiece is rotated, any chosen objective can be brought into position above the stage opening. The upper end of the tube holds the *ocular lens,* or eyepiece (a monocular scope has one; a binocular scope permits viewing with both eyes through two oculars).

6. Depending on the brand of microscope used, either the rotating nosepiece or the stage can be raised or lowered by *coarse* and *fine adjustment* knobs. These are located either above or below the stage. On some microscopes they are mounted as two separate knobs; on others they may be placed in tandem (see fig. 1.1) with the smaller fine adjustment extending from the larger coarse wheel. Locate the coarse adjustment on your microscope and rotate it gently, noting the upward or downward movement of the nosepiece or stage. The coarse adjustment is used to bring the objective down into position over any object on the stage, *while looking at it from the side* to avoid striking the object and thus damaging the expensive objective lens (fig. 1.3). The fine adjustment knob moves the tube to such a slight degree that movement cannot be observed from the side. It is used when one is viewing the object through the lenses to make the small adjustments necessary for a sharp, clear image.

Figure 1.3 When adjusting the microscope, the technologist observes the objective carefully to prevent breaking the slide and damaging the objective lens of the microscope. Photo by Bill Quinnell, Western Connecticut State University.

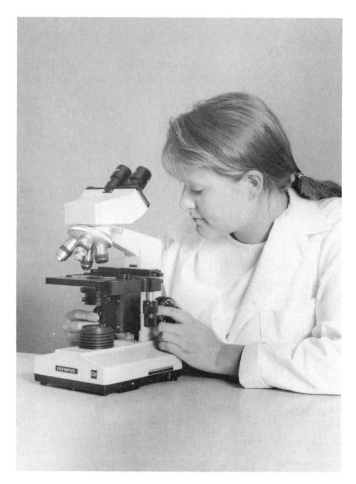

Turn the adjustment knobs *slowly* and *gently,* while paying attention to the relative positions of objective and object. Avoid bringing the objective *down* with the fine adjustment while viewing, because even this slight motion may force the lens against the object. Bring the lens safely down first with the coarse knob; then, while looking through the ocular, turn the fine knob to *raise* the lens until you have a clear view of the subject.

Rotating the fine adjustment too far in either direction may cause it to jam. If this should happen, *never attempt to force it;* call the instructor. To avoid jamming, gently locate the two extremes to which the fine knob can be turned, then bring it back to the middle of its span and keep it within one turn of this central position.

7. The *total magnification* achieved with the microscope depends on the combination of the *ocular* and *objective lens* used. Look at the ocular lens on your microscope. You will see that it is marked "10×," meaning that it magnifies 10 times.

Now look at the three objective lenses on the nosepiece. The short one is the *low-power* objective. Its metal shaft bears a "10×" mark, indicating that it gives tenfold magnification. When an object is viewed with the 10× objective combined with the 10× ocular, it is magnified 10 times 10, or ×100. Among your three objectives, this short one has the largest lens but the least magnifying power.

The other two objectives look alike in length, but one is an intermediate objective, called the *high-power* (or *high-dry*) *objective.* It may or may not have a colored ring on it. What magnification number is stamped on it? _____ What is the total magnification to be obtained when it is used with the ocular? _____

The third objective, which almost always has a colored ring, is called an *oil-immersion* objective. It has the smallest lens but gives the highest magnification of the three. (What is its magnifying number? _____ What total magnification will it provide together with the ocular? _____) This objective is the most useful of the three for the microbiologist because its high magnification permits clear viewing of all but the smallest microorganisms (viruses require an electron microscope). As its name implies, this lens must be immersed in a drop of oil placed on the object to be viewed. The oil improves the *resolution* of the magnified image, providing sharp detail even though it is greatly enlarged. The function of the oil is to prevent any scattering of light rays passing through the object and to direct them straight upward through the lens.

Notice that the higher the magnification used, the more intense the light must be, but the amount of illumination needed is also determined by the density of the object. For example, more light is needed to view stained than unstained preparations.

8. The *focal length* of an objective is directly proportional to the diameter of its lens. You can see this by comparing your three objectives when positioned as close to the stage as the coarse adjustment permits. First place the low-power objective in vertical position and bring it down with the coarse knob as far as it will go (gently!). The distance between the end of the objective, with its large lens, and the top of the stage is the focal length. Without moving the coarse adjustment, swing the high-power objective carefully into the vertical position, and note the much shorter focal length. Now, *with extreme caution,* bring the oil-immersion objective into place, making sure your microscope will permit this. If you think the lens will strike the stage or touch the condenser lens, *don't try it* until you have raised the nosepiece or lowered the stage (depending on your type of microscope) with the coarse adjustment. The focal length of the oil-immersion objective is between 1 and 2 mm, depending on the diameter of the lens it possesses (some are finer than others).

Never swing the oil-immersion objective into use position without checking to see that it will not make contact with the stage, the condenser, or the object being viewed. The oil lens alone is one of the most expensive and delicate parts of the microscope and must always be protected from scratching or other damage.

9. Take a piece of clean, soft *lens paper* and brush it lightly over the ocular and objective lenses and the top of the condenser. With subdued light coming through, look into the microscope. If you see specks of dust, rotate the ocular in its socket to see whether the dirt moves. If it does, it is on the ocular and should be wiped off more carefully. If you cannot solve the problem, call the instructor. *Never wipe the lenses with anything but clean, dry lens paper.* Natural oil from eyelashes, mascara, or other eye makeup can soil the oculars badly and seriously interfere with microscopy. Eyeglasses may scratch or be scratched by the oculars. If they are available, protective eyecups placed on the oculars prevent these problems. If not, you must learn how to avoid soiling or damaging the ocular lens.

10. *If oculars or objectives must be removed from the microscope for any reason, only the instructor or other delegated person should remove them. Inexperienced hands can do irreparable damage to a precision instrument.*

11. Because students in other laboratory sections may also use your assigned microscope, *you should examine the microscope carefully at the beginning of each laboratory session. Report any new defects or damage to the instructor immediately.*

B. Microscopic Examination of a Slide Preparation

1. Now that you are familiar with the parts and mechanisms of the microscope, you are ready to learn how to focus and use it to study microorganisms. The stained smear provided for you is a preparation of a yeast (*Candida albicans*) that is large enough to be seen easily even with the low-power objective. With the higher objectives, you will see that it has some interesting structures of different sizes and shapes that can be readily located as you study the effect of increasing magnification. You are not expected to learn the morphology of the organism at this point.

2. Place the stained slide securely in place on the stage, making certain it cannot slip or move. Position it so that light coming up through the condenser passes through the center of the stained area.

3. Bring the low-power objective into vertical position and lower it as far as it will go with the coarse adjustment, observing from the side.

4. Look through the ocular. If you have a monocular scope, keep both eyes open (you will soon learn to ignore anything seen by the eye not looking into the scope). If you have a binocular scope, adjust the two oculars horizontally to the width between your eyes until you have a single, circular field of vision. Now bring the objective slowly upward with the coarse adjustment until you can see small, blue objects in the field. Make certain the condenser is fully raised, and adjust the light to comfortable brightness with the iris diaphragm.

5. Use the fine adjustment knob to get the image as sharp as possible. Now move the slide slowly around, up and down, back and forth. The low-power lens should give you an overview of the preparation and enable you to select an interesting area for closer observation at the next higher magnification.

6. When you have selected an area you wish to study further, swing the high-dry objective into place. If you are close to sharp focus, make your adjustments with the fine knob. If the slide is badly out of focus with the new objective in place, look at the body tube and bring the lens down close to, but not touching, the slide. Then, looking through the ocular, adjust the lens slowly, first with the coarse adjustment, then with the fine, until you have a sharp focus. Notice the difference in magnification of the structures you see with this objective as compared with the previous one.

7. Without moving the slide and changing the field you have now seen at two magnifications, wait for the instructor to demonstrate the use of the oil-immersion objective.

8. Move the high-dry lens a little to one side and place a drop of oil on the slide, directly over the stage opening. With your eyes on the oil-immersion objective, bring it carefully into position making certain it does not touch the stage or slide. While still looking at the objective, gently lower the nosepiece (or raise the stage) until the tip of the lens is immersed in the oil but is not in contact with the slide. Look through the ocular and very slowly focus upward with the fine adjustment. Most microscopes are now *parfocal;* that is, the object remains in focus as you switch from one objective to another. In this case, the fine adjustment alone will bring the object into sharp focus. If you have trouble in finding the field or getting a clear image, ask the instructor for help. When you have a sharp focus, observe the difference in magnification obtainable with this objective as compared with the other two. It is about 2½ times greater than that provided by the high-power objective, and about 10 times more than that of the low-power lens.

9. Record your observations by drawing in each of the following circles several of the microbial structures you have seen, indicating their comparative size when viewed with each objective.

10. When you have finished your observations, remove the slide from the stage (taking care not to get oil on the high-dry lens) and gently clean the oil from the oil-immersion objective with a piece of dry lens paper.

Under each drawing, indicate the total magnification (TM) obtained by each objective combined with the ocular.

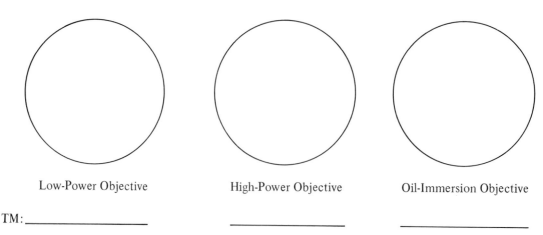

Low-Power Objective   High-Power Objective   Oil-Immersion Objective

TM: _____   _____   _____

C. Care and Handling of the Microscope

1. Always use both hands to carry the microscope, one holding the arm, one under the base (see fig. 1.2).
2. Before each use, examine the microscope carefully and report any unusual condition or damage.
3. Keep the oculars, objectives, and condenser lens clean. Use dry lens paper only.
4. At the end of each laboratory period in which the microscope is used, remove the slide from the stage, wipe away the oil on the oil-immersion objective, and place the low-power objective in vertical position.
5. Replace the dust cover, if available, and return the microscope to its box.

Table 1.1   Troubleshooting the Microscope

Problem	Possible Corrections
Insufficient light passing through ocular	Raise condenser
	Open iris diaphragm
	Check objective: is it locked in place?
Particles of dust or lint interfering with view of visual field	Wipe ocular and objective (*gently*) with clean lens paper
Moving particles in hazy visual field	Caused by bubbles in oil-immersion; check objective
	Make certain that the oil-immersion lens is in use, not the high-dry objective with oil on the slide
	Make certain the oil-immersion lens is in full contact with the oil

Questions

1. List the optical parts of the microscope. How does it achieve magnification? Resolution?

2. What is the function of the condenser?

3. What is the function of the iris diaphragm? To what part of the human eye would you compare it?

4. Why do you use oil on a slide to be examined with the oil-immersion objective?

5. What is the advantage of parfocal lenses?

6. If $5\times$ instead of $10\times$ oculars were used with the same objectives now on your microscope, what magnifications would be achieved?

EXERCISE 2   Handling and Examining Cultures

Reference: Morello, Mizer, Wilson, and Granato, Microbiology in Patient Care, 5th edition, 1994. Chapter 4.

Microscopic examination of microorganisms provides important information about their morphology but does not tell us much about their biological characteristics. To obtain such information, we need to observe microorganisms in *culture*. If we are to cultivate them successfully in the laboratory, we must provide them with suitable nutrients, such as protein components, carbohydrates, minerals, vitamins, and moisture in the right composition. This mixture is called a *culture medium* (plural, *media*). It may be prepared in liquid form, as a *broth,* or solidified with agar, a nonnutritive solidifying agent extracted from seaweed. *Agar media* may be used in tubes as a solid column (called a *deep*) or as *slants,* which have a greater surface area (see figs. 2.3 and 2.4). They are also commonly used in *petri dishes* (named for the German bacteriologist who designed them) or *plates,* as they are often called.

Solid media are essential for isolating and separating bacteria growing together in a specimen. If a mixture of bacteria is spread across the surface of an agar plate, individual organisms will multiply at individual sites until a visible aggregate called a *colony* is formed. One colony of a single species can then be separated from the rest and transferred to another medium, where it will grow as a *pure culture,* and can be studied as such.

The appearance of colonial growth on agar media can be very distinctive for individual species. Observation of the noticeable, gross features of colonies, that is, of their *colonial morphology,* is therefore very important. The color, density, consistency, surface texture, shape, and size of colonies all should be observed, for these features can provide clues as to the identity of an organism, although final identification cannot be made by morphology alone (fig. 2.1a).

In liquid media, some bacteria grow diffusely, producing uniform clouding, whereas others look very granular. Layering of growth at the top, center, or bottom of a broth tube reveals something of the organisms' oxygen requirements. Sometimes colonial aggregates are formed and the bacterial growth appears as small puff balls floating in the broth. Observation of such features can also be helpful in recognizing types of organisms (fig. 2.1b).

You must learn how to handle cultures aseptically. The organisms must not be permitted to contaminate the worker or the environment, and the cultures must not be contaminated with extraneous organisms. In this exercise, you will use cultures containing environmental organisms or organisms of low pathogenic potential. Nonetheless, you should handle them carefully to avoid contaminating yourself and your neighbors. Also, if you contaminate the cultures, your results will be spoiled. Before you begin, reread the opening paragraphs of Section I dealing with safety procedures and general laboratory directions (pp. 3–5).

Purpose	To make aseptic transfers of pure cultures and to examine them for important gross features
Materials	4 tubes of nutrient broth
	4 slants of nutrient agar
	One 24-hour slant culture of *Escherichia coli*
	One 24-hour slant culture of *Bacillus subtilis*
	One 24-hour slant culture of *Serratia marcescens* (pigmented)
	One 24-hour plate culture of *Serratia marcescens* (pigmented)
	Wire inoculating loop
	Bunsen burner (and matches)
	China-marking pencil or waterproof pen (or labels)
	A short ruler with millimeter markings

Figure 2.1 Examples of bacterial growth patterns. (a) Some colonial characteristics on agar media. Characteristics of the colony edges may be distinctive for many bacterial species. The shapes and elevations shown in the two rows of sketches are not intended to be matched. (b) Some growth patterns in broth media.

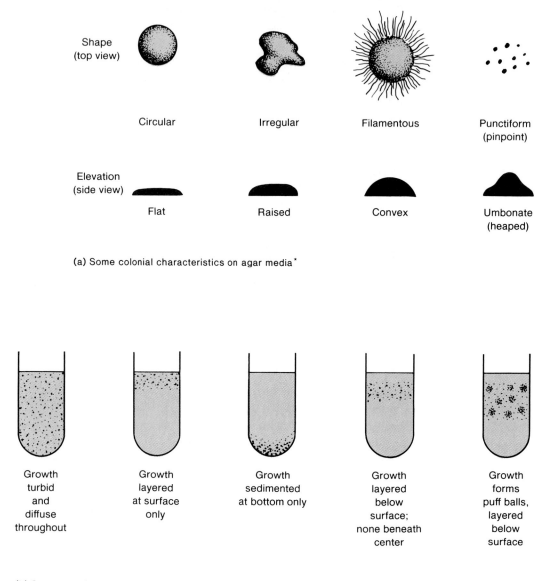

Shape (top view)

Circular   Irregular   Filamentous   Punctiform (pinpoint)

Elevation (side view)

Flat   Raised   Convex   Umbonate (heaped)

(a) Some colonial characteristics on agar media*

Growth turbid and diffuse throughout

Growth layered at surface only

Growth sedimented at bottom only

Growth layered below surface; none beneath center

Growth forms puff balls, layered below surface

(b) Some growth patterns in broth media

*Note: Shapes and elevations shown in this diagram are not intended to be matched.

Procedures

A. Transfer of a Slant Culture to a Nutrient Broth

1. The procedure will be demonstrated. Watch carefully and then do it yourself, following directions given.
2. Take up the inoculating loop by the handle and hold it as you would a pencil, loop down. Hold the wire in the flame of the Bunsen burner until it glows red (fig. 2.2). Remove loop from flame and hold it steady a few moments until cool. *Do not wave it around, put it down, or touch it to anything.*

Figure 2.2 Flaming the wire inoculating loop in the flame of a Bunsen burner.

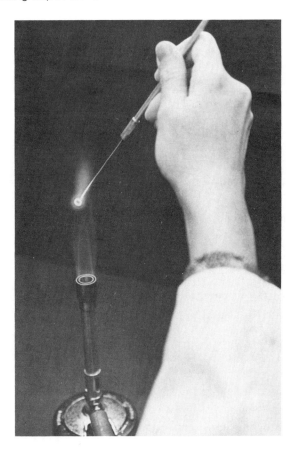

3. Pick up the slant culture of *Escherichia coli* with your left hand. Still holding the loop like a pencil, but more horizontally, in your right hand, use the little finger of the loop hand to remove the closure (cotton plug, slip-on, or screw cap) of the culture tube. Keep your little finger curled around this closure when it is free—*do not place it on the table* (fig. 2.3).

4. Pass the neck of the open tube rapidly through the Bunsen flame two or three times (don't overheat; if it is glass, it could crack or burn you later; if it is plastic, it could melt). This flaming sterilizes the air in and immediately around the mouth of the tube.

5. Insert the loop into the open tube (holding both horizontally). Touch the loop (*not the handle!*) to the growth on the slant and remove a loopful of culture. Don't dig the loop into the agar; merely scrape a small surface area gently.

6. Withdraw the loop slowly and steadily, being careful not to touch it to the mouth of the tube. Keep it steady, *and do not touch it to anything* (it's loaded!) while you replace the tube closure and put the tube back in the rack.

7. Still holding the loop steady in one hand, use the other hand to pick up a tube of sterile nutrient broth from the rack. Now remove the tube closure, as you did before, with the little finger of the loop hand (don't wave or jar the loop). Flame the neck of the tube; insert the loop into the tube and down into the broth. Gently rub the loop against the wall of the tube (don't agitate or splash the broth), making sure the liquid covers the area but does not touch the loop handle.

8. As you withdraw the loop, touch it to the inside wall of the tube (not the tube's mouth) to remove excess fluid from it. Pull it out without touching it again, flame the tube neck, replace the closure, and put the tube back in the rack.

Figure 2.3 Flaming an open culture tube to be inoculated. Notice that the tube is held almost horizontally. Its cap is tucked in the little finger of the right hand, which holds the inoculating loop.

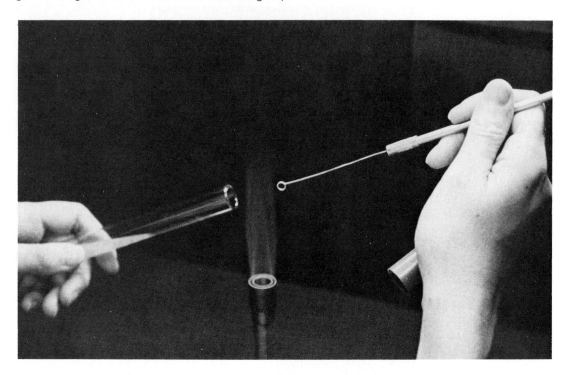

9. Now carefully flame the loop, holding it first in the coolest part of the flame (yellow), then in the hot blue cone until it glows. Be sure all of the wire is sterilized, but do not burn the handle. When the wire has cooled, the loop can be placed on the bench top.
10. Label the tube you have just inoculated with your name, the name of the organism, and the date.
11. Repeat steps 2 through 10 with each of the other two slant cultures (*Bacillus subtilis* and *Serratia marcescens*).

B. Transfer of a Slant Culture to a Nutrient Agar Slant

1. Start again with flaming the loop.
2. Pick up the slant culture of *E. coli,* open it, flame the neck of the tube, and take some growth up on the sterile loop.
3. When the culture tube has been flamed, closed, and replaced, pick up a sterile nutrient agar slant (keep the charged loop steady meantime). Open and flame it as before.
4. Introduce the charged loop into the fresh tube of agar, and without touching any surface, pass it down the tube to the *deep* end of the slant. Lightly touch the loop to the surface of the agar, swish it back and forth two or three times (don't dig up the agar), then zigzag it upward to the top of the slant. Lift the loop from the agar surface and withdraw it from the tube without touching the tube surfaces (fig. 2.4).
5. Flame, close, and replace the inoculated tube in the rack; then sterilize the loop as before.
6. Label the freshly inoculated tube with your name, the name of the organism, and the date.
7. Repeat steps 1 through 6 of procedure B with each of the other two slant cultures provided (*B. subtilis* and *S. marcescens*).

Basic Techniques of Microbiology

Figure 2.4 Streaking an agar slant with the loop.

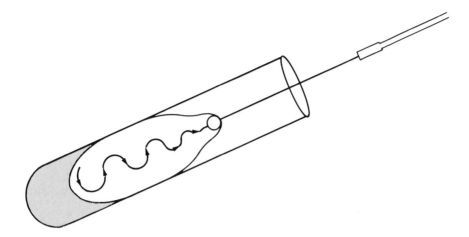

Figure 2.5 Opening a petri plate culture. The bottom is lifted out of the top, and the top is left lying face up on the bench.

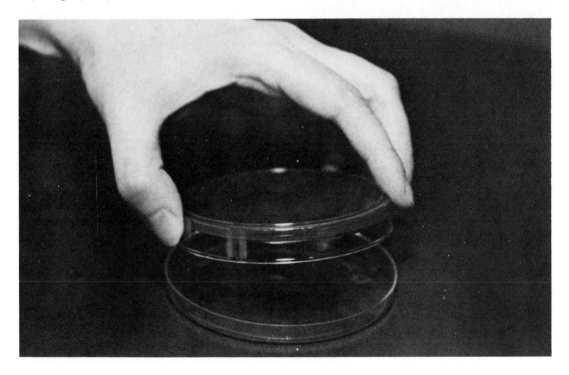

C. Transfer of a Single Bacterial Colony on a Plate Culture to a Nutrient Broth and a Nutrient Agar Slant

1. Start again with flaming the loop.
2. Hold the sterile, cooling loop in one hand and with the other hand turn the assigned plate culture of *Serratia marcescens* so that it is positioned with the bottom (smaller) part of the dish up. Lift this part of the dish with your free hand (fig. 2.5) and turn it so that you can clearly see isolated colonies of *S. marcescens* growing on the surface of the plated agar.

Figure 2.6 Selecting an isolated bacterial colony from a plate culture surface. The plate has been streaked so that single colonies have grown in well-separated positions and can easily be picked up.

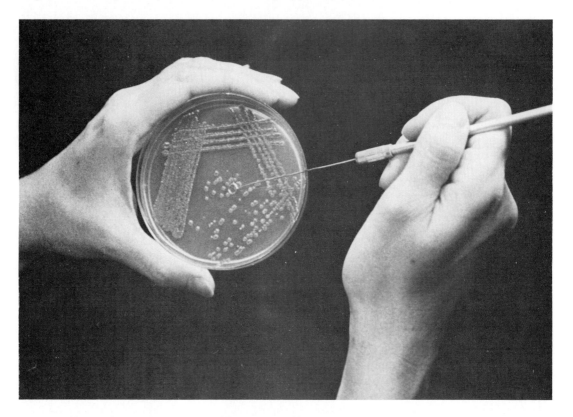

3. With the sterile, cool loop, touch the *surface* of one isolated bacterial colony (fig. 2.6). Withdraw the loop and replace the bottom part of the dish into the inverted top lying open on the table.
4. Now inoculate a sterile nutrient broth with the charged loop, as in procedure A, steps 7 through 10.
5. Flame the loop again, open the plate, pick another colony, close the plate, and inoculate a sterile agar slant as in procedure B, steps 4 through 6.

D. Incubation of Freshly Inoculated Cultures

1. Make certain all the broths (4) and slants (4) you have inoculated are properly and fully labeled.
2. Place your transferred cultures in an assigned rack in the incubator. The incubator temperature should be 35 to

   37°C. Record your reading of the incubator thermometer here. _____

E. Examination of Culture Growth

1. When you have finished making the culture transfers as directed, take a few minutes to look closely at the grown cultures assigned to you. In the Results section of this exercise, there is a blank form in which you can record information as to the appearance of these cultures, specifically: *size of colonies* (in mm), *color, density* (translucent? opaque?), *consistency* (creamy? dry? flaky?), *surface texture* (smooth? rough?), and *shape of colony* (margin even or serrated? flat? heaped?).
2. When the cultures you have made have grown out, record their appearance in broth or on slants, using the blank form in the Results section. Provide *all* the information the form requires, as in procedure E1.

Name _____ Class _____ Date _____

Results

Record your observations of all cultures in the following form:

Name of Organism	Appearance in Broth	Appearance on Slants or Plate				
		Size (mm)	Color	Density	Consistency	Colony Texture; Shape
Assigned cultures:						
Slant:						
1. _____	x	x				
2. _____	x	x				
3. _____	x	x				
Plate:		*				
4. _____	x					
Student cultures:						
1. _____		x				
2. _____		x				
3. _____		x				
4. _____		x				

*With your ruler, measure the diameter of the average colony appearing on the assigned plate culture by placing ruler on the *bottom* of the plate. Hold plate and ruler against the light to make your readings.

If you have made successful transfers and achieved pure cultures, the morphology of your cultures should match that of the ones you were assigned.

Questions

1. How would you determine whether culture media given to you are sterile before you use them?

2. What are the signs of growth in a liquid medium?

3. What is the purpose of wiping the laboratory bench top with disinfectant before you begin to handle cultures?

4. Why is the neck of a culture tube flamed when it is opened and flamed again before it is closed?

5. Why is it important to hold open culture tubes in a horizontal position?

6. Why can a single colony on a plate be used to start a pure culture?

7. Why is it important not to contaminate a pure culture?

8. What is meant by the term *colonial morphology?*

9. Why should long hair be controlled in a microbiology laboratory? Can you think of an actual patient-care situation that would call for its control for the same reason?

10. Name at least two kinds of solutions that may be administered to patients by intravenous injection and therefore must be sterile. How would you know if they were not sterile?

SECTION II

Microscopic Morphology of Microorganisms

EXERCISE 3 Hanging-Drop and Wet-Mount Preparations

Reference: Morello, Mizer, Wilson, and Granato, Microbiology in Patient Care, *5th edition, 1994. Chapter 4.*

Now that you have been oriented to some basic tools and methods used in microbiology, we shall begin our study of microorganisms by learning how to make preparations to study their morphology under the microscope.

The simplest method for examining living microorganisms is to suspend them in a fluid (water, saline, or broth) and prepare either a "hanging drop" or a simple "wet mount." The slide for a hanging drop is ground with a concave well in the center; the cover glass holds a drop of the suspension. When the cover glass is inverted over the well of the slide, the drop hangs from the glass in the hollow concavity of the slide (fig. 3.1, step 3). Microscopic study of such a wet preparation can provide useful information. Primarily, the method is used to determine whether or not an organism is motile, but it also permits an undistorted view of natural patterns of cell groupings and of individual cell shape. Hanging drop preparations can be observed for a fairly long time, because the drop does not dry up quickly. Wet-mounted preparations are used primarily to detect microbial motility rapidly. The fluid film is thinner than that of hanging-drop preparations and therefore the preparation tends to dry up more quickly, even when sealed.

Figure 3.1 Hanging-drop preparation using petroleum jelly to seal the cover glass to the slide.

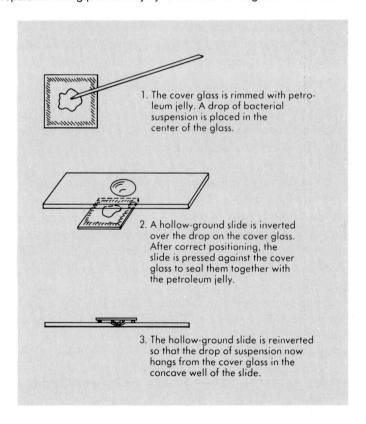

1. The cover glass is rimmed with petroleum jelly. A drop of bacterial suspension is placed in the center of the glass.

2. A hollow-ground slide is inverted over the drop on the cover glass. After correct positioning, the slide is pressed against the cover glass to seal them together with the petroleum jelly.

3. The hollow-ground slide is reinverted so that the drop of suspension now hangs from the cover glass in the concave well of the slide.

EXPERIMENT 3.1   Preparing a Hanging Drop

Purpose	To observe bacteria in a hanging drop, study their morphology, and determine their motility
Materials	24-hour broth culture of *Proteus vulgaris* mixed with a light suspension of yeast cells
	24-hour broth culture of *Staphylococcus epidermidis* mixed with a light suspension of yeast cells
	2 hollow-ground slides
	Several cover glasses
	Wire inoculating loop
	Bunsen burner
	China-marking pencil
	Petroleum jelly

Procedures

1. Take a cover glass and clean it thoroughly, making certain it is free of grease (the drop to be placed on it will not hang from a greasy surface). It may be dipped in alcohol and polished dry with tissue, or washed in soap and water, rinsed completely, and wiped dry. Place a thin film of petroleum jelly around the rim of the cover glass (fig. 3.1, step 1).

2. Take one hollow-ground slide and clean the well with a piece of dry tissue.

3. Gently shake the broth culture of *Proteus* until it is evenly suspended. Using the wire inoculating loop, the Bunsen flame, and good aseptic technique, remove a loopful of culture. Flame, close, and return the tube to the rack.

4. Place the loopful of culture in the center of the cover glass (do not spread it around). Flame the loop and put it down.

5. Hold the hollow-ground slide inverted, well down, over the cover glass (fig. 3.1, step 2), then press it down lightly so that the petroleum jelly adheres to the slide. Now turn the slide over. You should have a sealed wet mount, with the drop of culture hanging in the well (fig. 3.1, step 3).

6. Place the slide on the microscope stage, cover glass up. Start your examination with the low-power objective to find the focus. It is helpful to focus first on one edge of the drop, which will appear as a dark line. The light should be reduced with the iris diaphragm and, if necessary, by lowering the condenser. You should be able to focus easily on the yeast cells in the suspension. If you have trouble with the focus, ask the instructor for help.

7. Continue your examination with the high-dry and oil-immersion objectives (be very careful not to break the cover glass with the latter). Although the yeast cells will be obvious because of their larger size, look around them to observe the bacterial cells.

8. Make a hanging-drop preparation of the *Staphylococcus* culture, following the same procedures just described.

9. Record your observations of the size, shape, cell groupings, and motility of the two bacterial organisms in comparison to the yeast cells.

10. *Discard your slides in a container with disinfectant solution.*

Note: True, independent motility of bacteria depends on their possession of flagella. If so equipped, they can propel themselves with progressive, directional locomotion (often quite rapidly). This kind of active motion must be distinguished from the vibratory movement of organisms or other particles suspended in a fluid. The latter type of motion is called *Brownian movement* and is caused by the continuous, rapid oscillation of molecules in the fluid. Small particles of any kind, including bacteria (whether motile or not), are constantly bombarded by the vibration of the fluid molecules, and so are bobbed up and down, back and forth. Such movement is irregular and nondirectional and does not cause nonmotile organisms to change position with respect to other objects around them.

You must be careful not to mistake movement caused by currents in a liquid for true motility. If a wet mount is not well sealed or contains bubbles, air currents set up reacting fluid currents, and one sees organisms streaming along on a tide.

Results

1. Make drawings in the following circles to show the *shape* and *grouping* of each organism. Indicate below the circle whether it is *motile* or *nonmotile*. How does their size compare with that of the yeast cells in the preparation?

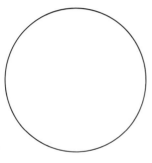

Proteus vulgaris

Motile _____

Nonmotile _____

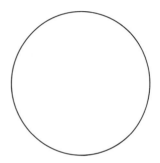

Staphylococcus epidermidis

Motile _____

Nonmotile _____

2. In the following left-hand circle, draw the path of a single bacterium having true motility. In the right-hand circle, draw the path of a single nonmotile bacterium.

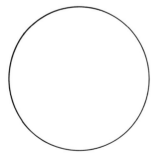

Path of a motile bacterium

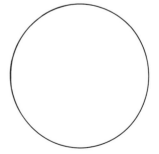

Path of a nonmotile bacterium

EXPERIMENT **3.2**   **Preparing a Wet Mount**

Purpose	To observe bacteria in a simple wet mount and determine their motility
Materials	24-hour broth culture of *Proteus vulgaris* mixed with a light suspension of yeast cells
	24-hour broth culture of *Staphylococcus epidermidis* mixed with a light suspension of yeast cells
	2 microscope slides
	Several cover glasses
	Capillary pipettes and pipette bulbs
	China-marking pencil
	Clear nail polish (optional)

Procedures

1. Using a pipette bulb, aspirate a small amount of the *Proteus* culture with a capillary pipette and place a *small* drop on a clean microscope slide (fig. 3.2, step 1).
2. Carefully place a clean cover glass (see Experiment 3.1 procedure 1 above) over the drop, trying to avoid bubble formation (fig. 3.2, step 2). The fluid should not leak out from under the edges of the cover glass. If it does, wait until it dries before sealing.
3. Seal around the edges of the coverslip with a thin film of clear nail polish (fig. 3.2, step 3). Be certain the nail polish is completely dry before examining the slide under the microscope. If you examine the slide quickly, you need not seal the coverslip.
4. Examine the preparation in the same manner as in Experiment 3.1 above, following procedures 6 through 10. Instead of focusing on the edge of the drop, however, you may find it helpful to focus first on the left-hand edge of the coverslip.

Figure 3.2 Wet-mount preparation.

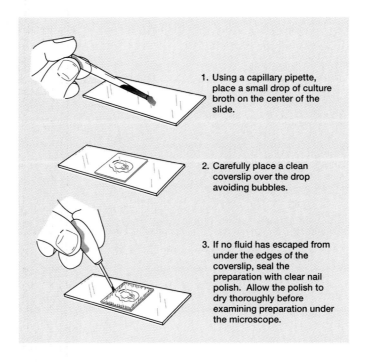

1. Using a capillary pipette, place a small drop of culture broth on the center of the slide.

2. Carefully place a clean coverslip over the drop avoiding bubbles.

3. If no fluid has escaped from under the edges of the coverslip, seal the preparation with clear nail polish. Allow the polish to dry thoroughly before examining preparation under the microscope.

Basic Techniques of Microbiology

Results

1. If you have not performed a hanging drop as in Experiment 3.1, make drawings in the circles above according to the directions in the results for that exercise.

2. If you have performed Experiment 3.1, complete the following chart.

	Hanging Drop	Wet Mount
	Motile (+ or −)	Motile (+ or −)
Proteus vulgaris		
Staphylococcus epidermidis		

Questions

1. How does true motility differ from Brownian movement?

2. What morphological structure is responsible for bacterial motility?

3. Why is a wet preparation discarded in disinfectant solution?

4. What is the value of a hanging-drop preparation?

5. What is the value of a wet-mount preparation?

EXERCISE 4 Simple Stains

Reference: Morello, Mizer, Wilson, and Granato, Microbiology in Patient Care, 5th edition, 1994. Chapter 4.

As we have seen in the previous exercise, wet mounts of bacterial cultures can be very informative, but they have limitations. Bacteria bounce about in fluid suspensions, with Brownian movement or true motility, and are difficult to visualize sharply. We can see their shapes and appreciate their activity under a cover glass, but it is difficult to form a complete idea of their morphology.

An important part of the problem is the minute size of bacteria. Because they are so small and have so little substance, they tend to be transparent, even when magnified in subdued light. The trick, then, is to find ways to stop their motion and tag their structures with something that will make them more visible to the human eye. Many sophisticated ways of doing this are known, but the simplest is to smear out a bacterial suspension, "fix" the organisms to the slide, then stain them with a visible dye (Koch and his coworkers first thought of this more than 100 years ago).

The best bacterial stains are *aniline dyes* (synthetic organic dyes made from coal-tar products). When they are used directly on fixed bacterial smears, the contours of bacterial bodies are clearly seen. These dyes are either *acidic, basic,* or *neutral* in reactivity. Acidic or basic stains are used primarily in bacteriologic work. The free ions of *acidic* dyes are anions (negatively charged) that combine with cations of a base in the stained cell to form a salt. *Basic* dyes possess cations (positively charged) that combine with an acid in the stained material to form a salt. Bacterial cells are rich in ribonucleic acid (contained in their abundant ribosomes) and therefore stain very well with basic dyes. *Neutral* stains are made by combining acidic and basic dyes. They are most useful for staining complex cells of higher forms because they permit differentiation of interior structures, some of which are basic, some acidic. Cells and structures that stain with basic dyes are said to be *basophilic.* Those that stain with acid dyes are termed *acidophilic.*

Stained bacteria can be measured for size and are classified by their shapes and groupings. Bacteria are so small that their size is most conveniently expressed in *micrometers* (symbol μm). A micrometer is a thousandth part of a millimeter, and 1/10,000 of a centimeter, or 1/25,400 of an inch. Bacteria vary in length and diameter, the smallest being about 0.5 to 1 μm long and approximately 0.5 μm in diameter, whereas the largest filamentous forms may be as long as 100 μm. Most of those you will see in this course are at the small end of the scale, measuring about 1 to 3 μm in length. Small as they are in reality, their images should loom large in your mind as the agents of infection in patients you will be caring for.

Bacteria have rigid cell walls and maintain a constant shape. Therefore, they can be classified on the basis of their form. Bacteria have three basic shapes. They may be *spherical, rod shaped,* or *spiraled* (fig. 4.1). A round bacterium is called a *coccus* (plural, *cocci*). A rod-shaped organism is called a *bacillus* (plural, *bacilli*) or simply a *rod.* A spiraled bacterium with at least two or three curves in its body is called a *spirillum* (plural, *spirilla*). Long sinuous organisms with many loose or tight coils are called *spirochetes.*

The patterns formed by bacterial cells grouping together as they multiply are often characteristic for individual bacterial genera or species. Cocci may occur in pairs (*diplococci*), chains (*streptococci*), clusters (*staphylococci*), or packets of four (*tetrads*), and are seldom found singly.

Rod-shaped bacteria (bacilli) generally occur as individual cells, but they may appear as end-to-end pairs (*diplobacilli*) or line up in chains (*streptobacilli*). Some species tend to *palisade,* that is, line up in bundles of parallel bacilli, or some may form V, X, or Y figures as they divide and split. Some may show great variation in their size and length (pleomorphism).

Spiraled bacteria occur singly and usually do not form group patterns. Examine colorplates 1–7 to see representative examples of bacterial morphology.

Figure 4.1 Basic shapes and arrangements of bacteria. (a) Cocci. 1. Diplococci (pairs); 2. Streptococci (chains); 3. Staphylococci (grapelike clusters); 4. Tetrads (packets of four). (b) Bacilli (rods). 1. Streptobacilli (chains); 2. Palisades; V, X, and Y figures, clubbing; 3. Endospore-forming bacilli (note endospores as small, round, hollow, unstained areas, within or at one end of bacillary bodies); 4. A bacillus showing pleomorphism (note varying widths and lengths). (c) Spirals. 1. Spirilla (short curved or spiraled forms with rigid bodies); 2. Spirochetes (long tightly or loosely coiled forms with sinuous flexible bodies).

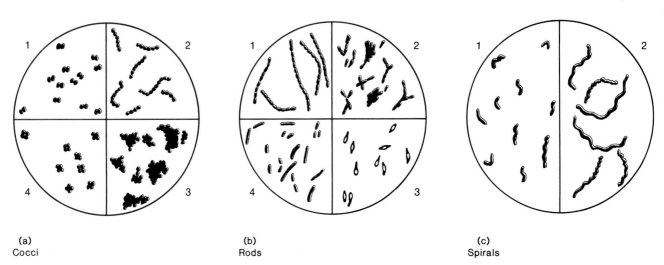

(a)
Cocci

(b)
Rods

(c)
Spirals

Purpose	To learn the value of simple stains in studying basic microbial morphology
Materials	24-hour agar culture of *Staphylococcus epidermidis*
	24-hour agar culture of *Bacillus subtilis*
	24-hour agar culture of *Escherichia coli*
	Prepared stained smear of a spiraled organism
	Loeffler's methylene blue
	Safranin
	Toothpicks
	Slides
	China-marking pencil

Procedures

1. Slides for microscopic smears must always be sparkling clean. They may be stored or dipped in alcohol and polished clean (free of grease) with a tissue or soft cloth.
2. Take three clean slides and with your marking pencil make a circle (about 1½ cm in diameter) in the center. At one end of the slide write the initials of one of the three assigned organisms (your three slides should read *Se, Bs,* and *Ec,* respectively).
3. Turn the slides over so that the unmarked side is up. (When slides are to be stained, wax pencil markings should always be placed on the underside so that the wax will not smear or wash off or run into the smear itself.)
4. Using your inoculating loop, place a loopful of water in the ringed area of the slide. Mix a *small* amount of bacteria in the water and spread it out.
5. Allow the smear to air dry. You should be able to see a thin white film. If not, add another loopful of water and more bacteria as in step 4.

Basic Techniques of Microbiology

6. Heat-fix the smear by passing the slide rapidly through the Bunsen flame three times.
7. Place the slides on a staining rack and flood them with Loeffler's methylene blue. Leave the stain on for three minutes.
8. Wash each slide gently with distilled water, drain off excess water, blot (do not rub) with bibulous paper, and let the slides dry completely in air.
9. Prepare two more slides as in steps 1, 2, and 3. Place a loopful of distilled water (or sterile saline) in the ringed area on each slide.
10. With the flat end of a toothpick, scrape some material from the surface of your teeth and around the gums. Emulsify the material in the drop of water on one slide. Repeat the procedure on the other slide.
11. Allow both slides to dry in air; then heat-fix them. Stain one with methylene blue for three minutes and another with safranin for three minutes.
12. Wash, drain, and dry the slides as in step 8.
13. Examine all slides, including the prepared stained smear assigned to you, with all three microscope objectives. Record your results in the following table.

Results

Organism in Broth Culture	Stain	Color	Coccus Rod Spiral	Cell Grouping	Diagram
S. epidermidis					
B. subtilis					
E. coli					
Prepared smear					

Draw the organisms you saw in the scraping from your teeth.

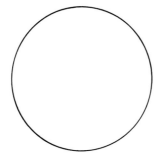

Describe the results you obtained with the two stains used. Which provided the sharpest view?

Questions

1. Define *acidic* and *basic dyes.* What is the purpose of each?

2. What is the purpose of flaming a slide that is to be stained?

3. Why are specimens to be stained suspended in *sterile* saline or *distilled* water?

4. Which of the microscope objectives is most satisfactory for studying bacteria? Why?

5. How does a stained preparation compare with a hanging drop for studying the morphology and motility of bacteria?

6. List at least three types of bacteria whose names reflect their shapes and arrangements, and state the meaning of each name.

7. List and define the basic shapes of bacteria. What are the dimensions of an average bacillus in micrometers? In centimeters?

8. For what reason do we need to stain bacteria?

9. Examine colorplates 1–7 and describe the morphology of the bacteria in each one.

SECTION III

Differential Stains

EXERCISE 5 Gram Stain

*Reference: Morello, Mizer, Wilson, and Granato, Microbiology in Patient Care, 5th edition, 1994.
Chapter 4.*

The simple staining procedure performed in Exercise 4 makes it possible to see bacteria clearly, but it does not distinguish between organisms of similar morphology.

In 1884, a Danish pathologist, Christian Gram, discovered a method of staining bacteria with pararosaniline dyes. Using two dyes in sequence, each of a different color, he found that bacteria fall into two groups. The first group retains the color of the primary dye: crystal violet (these are called *gram-positive*). The second group loses the first dye when washed in a decolorizing solution but then takes on the color of the second dye, a *counterstain,* such as safranin or carbol fuchsin (these are called *gram-negative*). An iodine solution is used as a *mordant* (a chemical that fixes a dye in or on a substance by combining with the dye to form an insoluble compound) for the first stain.

The exact mechanism of action of this staining technique is not clearly understood. However, it is known that differences in the biochemical composition of bacterial cell walls parallel differences in their Gram-stain reactions. Gram-positive bacterial walls are rich in peptidoglycans (protein-sugar complexes) that enable cells to resist decolorization. Gram-negative bacterial walls have a high concentration of lipids (fats) that dissolve in the decolorizer (alcohol or acetone or a mixture of these) and are washed away with the crystal violet. The decolorizer thus prepares gram-negative organisms for the counterstain.

The Gram stain is one of the most useful tools in the microbiology laboratory and is used universally. In the diagnostic laboratory, it is used not only to study microorganisms in cultures, but it is also applied to smears made directly from clinical specimens. Direct, Gram-stained smears are read promptly to determine the relative numbers and morphology of bacteria in the specimen. This information is valuable to the physician in planning the patient's treatment before culture results are available. It is also valuable to microbiologists, who can plan their culture procedures based on their knowledge of the bacterial forms they have seen in the specimen.

The numerous modifications of Gram's original method are based on the concentration of the dyes, length of staining time for each dye, and composition of the decolorizer. Hucker's modification, to be followed in this exercise, is commonly used today. The choice of decolorizing agent depends on the speed wanted to accomplish this step. The slowest agent, 95% ethyl alcohol, is used in this exercise to permit the student to gain experience with decolorization. Acetone is the fastest decolorizer, while an equal mixture of 95% ethyl alcohol and acetone acts with intermediate speed. The acetone-alcohol combination is probably the most popular in diagnostic laboratories.

Purpose	To learn the Gram-stain technique and to understand its value in the study of bacterial morphology
Materials	24-hour broth or agar culture of the following organisms:

        Staphylococcus epidermidis
        Enterococcus faecalis
        Neisseria sicca
        Saccharomyces cerevisiae (yeast)
        Bacillus subtilis
        Escherichia coli
        Proteus vulgaris
Specimen of simulated pus from a postoperative wound infection
Hucker's crystal violet
Gram's iodine
Ethyl alcohol, 95%
Safranin
Slides
China-marking pencil and slide labels

Procedures

1. Prepare a fixed smear of each culture and one of the simulated clinical specimen. On the underside of each slide, make a penciled code mark so that you can identify the slides after staining.
2. Stain each smear by the following procedures (this is Hucker's modification of the Gram stain):
    a. Flood slide with crystal violet. Allow to stand for one minute (check with instructor; time varies with different batches of stain).
    b. Wash off with tap water.
    c. Flood with Gram's iodine (a mordant). Leave for one minute.
    d. Wash off with tap water.
    e. Decolorize with alcohol (95%) until no more color washes off (usually 10–20 seconds). This is a most critical step. Be careful not to overdecolorize, as many gram-positive organisms may lose the violet stain easily and thus appear to be gram-negative after they are counterstained.
    f. Apply safranin (the counterstain) for one minute.
    g. Wash off with tap water.
    h. Drain and blot gently with bibulous paper.
3. When slides are dry, label them as shown:

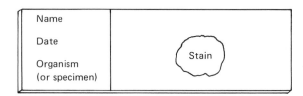

4. Examine all slides under oil with the oil-immersion objective.
5. Record observations in table under Results.
6. Examine colorplates 1–6 and 10 and note which bacteria are gram-positive or gram-negative.

Results

Name of Organism	Color	Gram-Stain Reaction	Diagram
Broth or agar cultures			
Pus specimen: Describe type(s) of organisms seen			

Questions

1. What is the function of the iodine solution in the Gram stain? If it were omitted, how would staining results be affected?

2. What is the purpose of the alcohol solution in the Gram stain?

3. What counterstain is used? Why is it necessary? Could colors other than red be used?

4. On the basis of Gram reaction, can you distinguish species of:

Staphylococcus and *Streptococcus?* _____

Staphylococcus and *Neisseria?* _____

Escherichia and *Proteus?* _____

Escherichia and *Bacillus?* _____

5. What is the size of staphylococci in micrometers? In centimeters?

6. What is the advantage of the Gram stain over the simple stain?

7. In what kind of clinical situation would a direct smear report from the laboratory be of urgent importance?

8. What is the current theory about the mechanism of the Gram-stain reaction?

9. Describe at least two conditions in which an organism might stain gram variable.

EXERCISE 6 Acid-Fast Stain

Reference: Morello, Mizer, Wilson, and Granato, Microbiology in Patient Care, 5th edition, 1994. Chapters 4, 12, 19.

Members of the bacterial genus *Mycobacterium* contain large amounts of lipid (fatty) substances within their cell walls. These fatty waxes resist staining by ordinary methods. Because this genus contains species that cause important human diseases (the agent of tuberculosis is a *Mycobacterium*), the diagnostic laboratory must use special stains to reveal them in clinical specimens or cultures (see also Exercise 29).

When these organisms are stained with a basic dye, such as carbolfuchsin, applied with heat or in a concentrated solution, the stain can penetrate the lipid cell wall and reach the cell cytoplasm. Once the cytoplasm is stained, it resists decolorization, even with harsh agents such as acid-alcohol, which cannot dissolve and penetrate beneath the mycobacterial lipid wall. Under these conditions of staining, the mycobacteria are said to be *acid fast* (see colorplate 8). Other bacteria whose cell walls do not contain high concentrations of lipid are readily decolorized by acid-alcohol after staining with carbolfuchsin and are said to be *nonacid-fast*. One medically important genus, *Nocardia*, contains species that are *partially acid fast*. They resist decolorization with a weak (1%) sulfuric acid solution, but lose the carbolfuchsin dye when treated with acid-alcohol. In the acid-fast technique, a counterstain is used to demonstrate whether or not the fuchsin has been decolorized within cells and the second stain taken up.

The original technique for applying carbolfuchsin with heat is called the *Ziehl-Neelsen stain,* named after the two bacteriologists who developed it in the late 1800s. The later modification of the technique employs more concentrated carbolfuchsin reagent rather than heat to ensure stain penetration and is known as the *Kinyoun stain.*

Purpose	To learn the acid-fast technique and to understand its value when used to stain a clinical specimen
Materials	A young slant culture of *Mycobacterium phlei* (a saprophyte)
	24-hour broth culture of *Bacillus subtilis*
	A sputum specimen simulating that of a 70-year-old man from a nursing home, admitted to the hospital with chest pain and bloody sputum
	Gram-stain reagents
	Kinyoun's carbolfuchsin
	Acid-alcohol solution
	Methylene blue
	Slides
	Diamond glass-marking pencil
	China-marking pencil
	2 × 3-cm filter paper strips
	Slide rack
	Forceps

Procedures

1. Prepare two heat-fixed smears of each culture and two of the simulated sputum. In practice, the smears are heat fixed at 65 to 75° C to be certain any tuberculosis bacilli present are killed. To make smears of the agar slant culture, first place a drop of water on the slide, and then emulsify a small amount of the colonial growth in this drop.
2. Ring and code one slide of each pair with your china-marking pencil, as usual.
3. The other slide of each pair must be ringed and coded with a diamond pencil. This device scratches the glass indelibly, so that the marks remain even during the prolonged staining process.
4. Gram stain the set of slides marked with a wax pencil.
5. Stain the diamond-scratched slides by the Kinyoun technique, as follows:
   a. Place the slides on a slide rack extended over a metal staining tray, if available.
   b. Cover smear with a 2 X 3 cm piece of filter paper to hold the stain on the slide and to filter out any undissolved dye crystals.
   c. Flood the slide with concentrated carbolfuchsin solution and allow to stand for five minutes.
   d. Use forceps to remove filter paper strips from slides and place the strips in a discard container. Rinse slides with water and drain.
   e. Cover smears with acid-alcohol solution and allow them to stand for two minutes.
   f. Rinse again with water and drain.
   g. Flood smear with methylene blue and counterstain for one to two minutes.
   h. Rinse, drain, and air dry.
6. Examine all slides under oil immersion and record observations under Results.

Results

Name of Organism	Visible in Gram Stain* (Yes, No)	Gram-Stain Reaction (If Visible)	Visible in Acid-Fast Stain (Yes, No)	Color in Acid-Fast Stain	Acid-Fast Reaction (If Visible)
Cultures					
Sputum specimen (describe organism)					

*Note: Some saprophytic mycobacteria may stain weakly gram positive or appear beaded in Gram-stained smears.

Basic Techniques of Microbiology

Questions

1. What is a differential stain? Name two examples of such stains.

2. Is a Gram stain an adequate substitute for an acid-fast stain? Why?

3. When is it appropriate to ask the laboratory to perform an acid-fast stain?

4. In light of the clinical history (p. 41) and your observations of the Gram and acid-fast smears, what is your tentative diagnosis of the patient's illness? How should this preliminary laboratory diagnosis be confirmed?

5. Are saprophytic mycobacteria acid fast?

6. Does the presence of acid-fast organisms in a clinical specimen always suggest serious clinical disease?

7. How should the acid-fast stain of a sputum specimen from a patient with suspected pulmonary *Nocardia* infection be performed?

EXERCISE 7 Special Stains

Reference: Morello, Mizer, Wilson, and Granato, Microbiology in Patient Care, *5th edition, 1994. Chapters 2, 4.*

Some bacteria have characteristic surface structures (such as *capsules* or *flagella*) and internal components (e.g., *endospores*) which may have taxonomic value for their identification. When it is necessary to demonstrate whether or not a particular organism possesses a capsule, is flagellated, or forms endospores, special staining techniques must be used.

Many bacteria possess a capsule, but it is often not visible. A few pathogenic species, however, such as *Streptococcus pneumoniae, Klebsiella pneumoniae,* and *Clostridium perfringens,* have well-developed capsules that contribute to virulence by protecting the organisms from host defense mechanisms, particularly phagocytosis. Furthermore, capsular substances are often antigenic, providing the bacterial cell with specific immunologic properties by which they may be identified. Different strains of pneumococci, klebsiellae, or other encapsulated bacteria, for example, can be identified serologically, by means of the *quellung reaction.* In this test, when an organism of a particular antigenic type is mixed with its specific antiserum, capsular antigen reacts with antibody at the cell surface. When the organism is viewed through the microscope as this reaction occurs, the capsule appears to swell as it becomes much more distinct and demarcated (see colorplate 9). Capsules can also be visualized microscopically by using a simple, nonspecific *negative staining technique.* For this preparation, materials such as India ink or nigrosin are first applied to a suspension of bacterial cells placed on a glass slide. These agents do not penetrate the cells but outline their surface structures. After drying, the slide preparation is stained with safranin, a dye that does penetrate the cells and stains them. When viewed under the microscope after this treatment, the bacteria are pink, while their capsules appear as clear, unstained zones surrounding them, their outlines demarcated against the black background provided by the India ink or nigrosin. *Direct staining methods* can also be used to demonstrate bacterial capsules. In the Hiss method, for example, a bacterial suspension is placed on a glass slide, allowed to dry, and heat-fixed. The smear is then flooded with a 1% aqueous solution of crystal violet, gently steamed, and rinsed with copper sulfate (20% aqueous solution). Under the microscope, the capsules appear as faintly stained blue halos surrounding dark blue to purple cells.

Bacterial flagella are tiny hairlike organelles of locomotion. Originating in the cytoplasm beneath the cell wall, they extend beyond the cell, usually equaling or exceeding it in length. Their fine protein structure requires special staining techniques for demonstrating them with the light microscope. Since not all bacteria possess flagella, their presence, numbers, and pattern or arrangement on the cell may provide clues to identification of species (fig. 7.1). For example, *Vibrio cholerae* and some species of *Pseudomonas* have a single polar flagellum at one end of the cell (they are said to be *monotrichous*), some spirillae display bipolar tufts of flagella (the arrangement is called *lophotrichous*), while many *Proteus* species have multiple flagella surrounding their cells (in a *peritrichous* pattern). Some flagellar stains employ rosaniline dyes and a mordant, applied to a bacterial suspension fixed in formalin and spread across a glass slide. The formalin links to or "fixes" the flagellar and other surface protein of the cells. The dye and mordant then precipitate around these "fixed" surfaces, enlarging their diameters, and making flagella visible when viewed under the microscope. In another method, a ferric-tannate mordant and a silver nitrate solution are applied to a bacterial suspension. The resulting dark precipitate that forms on the bacteria and their flagella allows them to be easily visualized under the microscope. This silver-plating technique is also used to stain the very slender spirochetes.

Among bacteria, endospore formation is most characteristic of two genera, *Bacillus* and *Clostridium.* The process of sporulation involves the condensation of vital cellular components within a thick, double-layered wall enclosing a round or ovoid inner body. The activities of the vegetative (actively growing) cell slow down, and it loses moisture as the endospore is formed. Gradually, the empty bacterial shell falls away. The remaining endospore is highly resistant to environmental influences, representing a resting, protective stage. Most disinfectants cannot permeate it, and it resists the lethal effects of drying, sunlight, ultraviolet radiation, and boiling. It can be killed when dry heat is applied at high temperatures or for long periods, by steam heat under pressure (in the autoclave), or by special sporicidal (endospore-killing) disinfectants. Because bacterial endospore walls are not readily permeated by materials in solution, the inner contents of the endospores are not easily stained by ordinary bacterial dyes. When sporulating bacteria are Gram stained,

Figure 7.1 Arrangements of bacterial flagella.

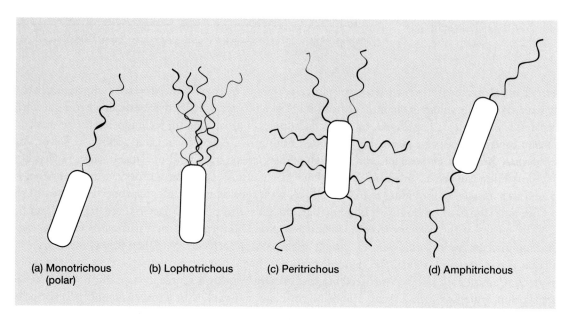

(a) Monotrichous (polar)   (b) Lophotrichous   (c) Peritrichous   (d) Amphitrichous

the endospores forming within the vegetative cells appear as empty holes in the bacterial bodies (see colorplate 10). Depending on their location within the cell, the endospores are referred to as terminal (at the very end of the vegetative cell), subterminal (near, but not at, the end of the cell), or central. Free endospores are invisible when stained with the Gram stain or appear as faint pink rings. To demonstrate the inner contents of bacterial endospores, you must use a special staining technique that can drive a dye through the endospore coat.

EXPERIMENT 7.1   Staining Bacterial Endospores (Schaeffer-Fulton Method)

Purpose	To learn a technique for staining bacterial endospores
Materials	3- to 5-day old agar slant culture of *Bacillus subtilis* 24-hour old slant culture of *Staphylococcus epidermidis* Malachite green solution Safranin solution Slides Diamond glass-marking pencil Slide rack 500-ml beaker Tripod with asbestos mat Forceps

Figure 7.2 A simple method for applying heat when staining smears, using the endospore stain technique.

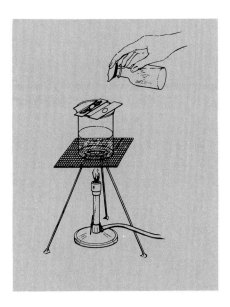

Procedures

1. Place a drop of water on a slide. Emulsify a small amount of each of the slant cultures in the same drop of water.
2. Ring and code the slide with the diamond marking pencil.
3. Stain the slide by the endospore stain as follows:
   a. Place the slides on a slide rack extended across a beaker of boiling water held on a tripod (an electric burner may be used instead of a Bunsen burner). An asbestos mat should protect the beaker from the Bunsen flame beneath (fig. 7.2).
   b. Flood slide with malachite green and allow to steam gently for 3 to 5 minutes. The stain itself should not boil; if it does, reduce the heat. If the stain appears to be evaporating and drying too rapidly, add a little more. Keep the slide flooded.
   c. Allow the slide to cool slightly, then use forceps to drain the slide over a sink or staining tray and rinse with water for about 30 seconds until no more green washes out.
   d. Counterstain the preparation with safranin for 30 seconds, then rinse again with tap water. Blot or air-dry the slide.
   e. Examine the smear under the oil-immersion objective and record your observations under Results.

Results

1. In the circle below, make a sketch of your microscopic observations. Note the difference between the staining properties of the staphylococci and the endospores. Use colored pencils if they are available. Indicate the color of the spores in contrast to the vegetative cells.

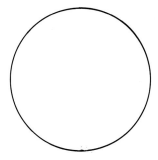

What is the location of the endospore within the bacterial cell (e.g., terminal, subterminal, central)? _____

_____

Purpose	To examine microorganisms stained by various methods to demonstrate their flagella and capsules
Materials	Prepared slides stained to reveal: Bacterial flagella (monotrichous, lophotrichous, and peritrichous or other patterns of arrangement) Bacterial capsules (direct or negative staining)

Procedures

1. Examine the prepared slides and make drawings of your observations.
2. Review assigned reading and be prepared to discuss the morphological classification of bacteria.

Results

Record and diagram your observations:

Bacterial endospores

Color of

Endospores _____

Bacillus vegetative cells ____

Staphylococcus cells _____

Bacterial flagella

Color of

Flagella _____

Cells _____

Background _____

Bacterial capsules

Color of

Capsules _____

Cells _____

Background _____

Describe the arrangement of flagella you observed: _____

_____

Questions

1. Why must special stains be used to visualize bacterial capsules, flagella, and endospores?

2. Why is it important to know whether or not bacterial cells possess capsules, flagella, or endospores?

3. What do endospore stains have in common with the Ziehl-Neelsen acid-fast stain?

4. Is bacterial sporulation a reproductive process? Explain.

5. Why is it important to determine the location of the endospore within the bacterial cell?

6. Can you relate endospore staining to endospore survival in hospital or other environments?

7. What is a negative stain?

8. Describe a flagella stain and explain the principle of its action.

9. Compare the usefulness of a flagella stain with that of the hanging-drop or wet-mount preparation.

10. What is the quellung reaction? How might it be used to rapidly identify certain bacteria directly in clinical specimens?

11. Of what value is a capsule to a microorganism?

SECTION IV

Cultivation of Microorganisms

EXERCISE 8 Culture Media

Reference: Morello, Mizer, Wilson, and Granato, Microbiology in Patient Care, 5th edition, 1994. Chapter 4.

Knowing the microscopic morphology and staining characteristics of a microorganism present in a clinical specimen, the microbiologist can make appropriate decisions as to how it should be cultivated and what biological properties must be demonstrated to identify it fully.

First, a suitable culture medium must be provided, and it must contain the nutrients essential for the growth of the microorganism to be studied (see Exercise 2). Most media designed for the initial growth and isolation of microorganisms are rich in protein components derived from animal meats. Many bacteria are unable to break down proteins to usable forms and must be provided with extracted or partially degraded protein materials (peptides, proteoses, peptones, amino acids). Meat extracts, or partially cooked meats, are the basic nutrients of many culture media. Some carbohydrate and mineral salts are usually added as well. Such basal media may then be supplemented, or *enriched,* with blood, serum, vitamins, other carbohydrates and mineral salts, or particular amino acids as needed or indicated.

In this exercise, we will prepare a basic nutrient broth medium and also a nutrient agar from commercially available dehydrated stock mixtures containing all necessary ingredients except water. The term *nutrient broth* (or *agar*) refers specifically to basal media prepared from *meat extracts,* with a few other basic ingredients, but lacking special enrichment. We will also see how liquid and agar media are appropriately dispensed in flasks, bottles, or tubes for sterilization before use, and how a sterile agar medium is then poured aseptically into petri dishes.

Purpose	To learn how culture media are prepared for use in the microbiology laboratory
Materials	Dehydrated nutrient agar
	Dehydrated nutrient broth
	A balance, and weighing papers
	A 1-liter Erlenmeyer flask, cotton plugged or screw capped
	A 1-liter glass beaker
	A 1-liter graduated cylinder
	Glass stirring rods (at least 10 cm long)
	10-ml pipettes (cotton plugged)
	Test tubes (screw capped or cotton plugged)
	Petri dishes
	Aspiration device for pipetting

Procedures

1. Read the label on a bottle of dehydrated nutrient *agar.* It specifies the amount of dehydrate required to make 1 liter (1,000 ml) of medium. Calculate the amount needed for ½ liter and weigh out this quantity.
2. Place 500 ml of distilled water in an Erlenmeyer flask. Add the weighed, dehydrated agar while stirring with a glass rod to prevent lumping.
3. Set the flask on a tripod over an asbestos mat. Using a Bunsen flame, *slowly* bring the rehydrated agar to a boil. Stir often. An electric hot plate may be used instead of a Bunsen burner.
4. When the agar mixture is completely dissolved, remove the flask from the flame or hot plate, close it with the cotton plug or cap, and give it to the instructor to be sterilized in the autoclave.
5. While the agar flask is being sterilized, prepare 500 ml of nutrient *broth,* adding the weighed dehydrate to the water in a beaker for reconstitution and dissolution.

Figure 8.1 Flaming the mouth of a flask of melted agar that is to be plated.

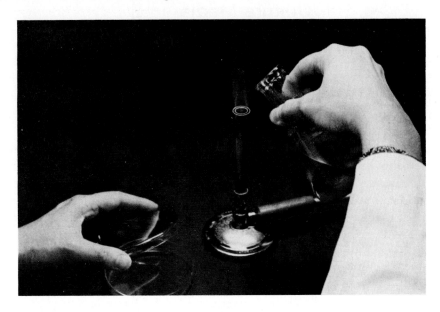

6. Bring the reconstituted broth to a boil, *slowly*. When fully dissolved, remove from flame and allow to cool a bit.
7. The instructor will demonstrate the use of the pipetting device. *Do not pipette by mouth.* Using a pipette, dispense 5-ml aliquots of the broth into test tubes (plugged or capped). The instructor will collect the tubes and sterilize them.
8. When the flask of sterilized agar is returned to you, allow it to cool to about 50°C (the agar should be warm and melted, but not too hot to handle in its flask). Remove the plug or cap with the little finger of your right hand and continue to hold it until you are sure it won't have to be returned to the flask. Flame the open mouth of the flask (fig. 8.1), and quickly pour the melted, sterile agar into a series of petri dishes. The petri dish tops are lifted with the left hand, and the bottoms are filled to about one-third capacity with melted agar. Replace each petri dish top as the plate is poured. When the plates are cool (agar solidified), invert them to prevent condensing moisture from accumulating on the agar surfaces.
9. Place inverted agar plates and tubes of sterilized nutrient broth (cooled after their return to you) in the 35°C incubator. They should be incubated for at least 24 hours to ensure their sterility before you use them in the next exercise.

Results

After at least 24 hours of incubation at 35°C, do your prepared plates and broths appear to be sterile?

_____

Record your observation of their physical appearance:

Plates: _____

_____

Broths: _____

Questions

1. Define a *culture medium*.

2. Discuss some of the physical and chemical factors involved in the *composition*, and in the *preparation*, of a culture medium:

   Nutrient ingredients: _____

   _____

   _____

   pH and buffering: _____

   _____

   Heat (to reconstitute): _____

   Heat (to sterilize): _____

   _____

   Other: _____

   _____

3. At what temperature does agar solidify? _____

   At what temperature does agar melt? _____

4. What would happen to plates poured with agar that is too hot? _____

   _____

   Could they be used? _____

5. What would happen to plates poured with agar that is too cool? _____

   Could they be used? _____

6. Why are culture media sterilized prior to use?

7. Discuss the relative value of broth and agar media in *isolating* bacteria from mixed cultures.

8. Are nutrient broths and agars, as you have prepared them, suitable for supporting growth of all microorganisms pathogenic for humans? Explain your answer.

EXERCISE 9 Pure Culture Technique

Reference: Morello, Mizer, Wilson, and Granato, Microbiology in Patient Care, 5th edition, 1994. Chapter 4.

The skin and many mucosal surfaces of the human body support large numbers of microorganisms that comprise the normal, or indigenous, flora. When clinical specimens are collected from these surfaces and cultured, any pathogenic microorganisms being sought must be recognized among, and isolated from, other harmless organisms. Colonies of the pathogenic species must be picked out of the *mixed* culture and grown in isolated *pure* culture. The microbiologist can then proceed to identify the isolated organism by examining its biochemical and immunological properties. Pure culture technique is critical to successful, accurate identification of microorganisms (see colorplates 11–13).

Purpose	A. To isolate pure cultures from a specimen containing mixed flora
	B. To culture and study the normal flora of the mouth
Materials	Nutrient agar plates*
	Blood agar plates
	Sterile swabs
	A mixed broth culture containing *Serratia marcescens* (pigmented), *Escherichia coli,* and *Staphylococcus epidermidis*
	A demonstration plate culture made from this broth, showing colonies isolated by the streak dilution technique
	Glass slides
	Gram-stain reagents

*If the plates you prepared in Exercise 8 are sterile and in good condition, they may be used in this experiment.

Procedures

A. Streaking a Mixed Broth Culture for Colony Isolation

1. Make certain the contents of the broth culture tube are evenly mixed.
2. Place a loopful of broth culture on the surface of a nutrient agar plate, near but not touching the edge. With the loop flat against the agar surface, lightly streak the inoculum back and forth over approximately one-eighth the area of the plate; do not dig up the agar (fig. 9.1, area A).
3. Flame the loop and let it cool in air.
4. Rotate the open plate in your left hand so that you can streak a series of four lines back and forth, each passing through the inoculum and extending across one side of the plate (fig. 9.1, area B).
5. Flame the loop again and let it cool in air.
6. Rotate the plate and streak another series of four lines, each crossing the end of the last four streaks and extending across the adjacent side of the plate (fig. 9.1, area C).
7. Rotate the plate and repeat this parallel streaking once more (fig. 9.1, area D).
8. Finally, make a few streaks in the untouched center of the plate (fig. 9.1, area E). *Do not touch the original inoculum.*
9. Incubate the plate (inverted) at 35°C.

Figure 9.1 Diagram of streak dilution technique. The goal is to thin the numbers of bacteria growing in each successive area of the plate as it is rotated and streaked so that isolated colonies will appear in sections D and E.

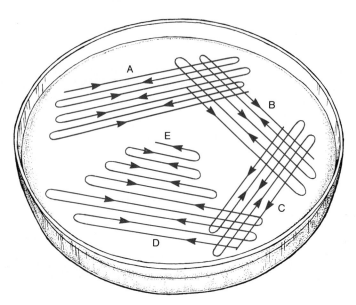

B. Taking a Culture from the Mouth

1. Rotate a sterile swab over the surface of your tongue and gums.
2. Roll the swab over a small 1½-cm square of surface of a blood agar plate, near but not touching one edge (see fig. 9.1, area A). Rotate the swab fully in this area.
3. Discard the swab in a container of disinfectant.
4. Using an inoculating loop, streak the plate by the streak dilution technique as in figure 9.1.
5. Incubate the plate (inverted) at 35°C.

Results

A. Examination of Plate Streaked from Mixed Broth Culture

1. Examine the incubated nutrient agar plate carefully. Compare your streaking with that illustrated in figure 9.2a and b. Make a drawing showing the intensity of growth in each streaked area.

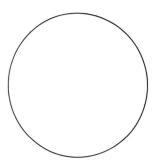

Basic Techniques of Microbiology

Figure 9.2 Plate streaking. (a) Streak dilution technique. Notice how this technique is designed to yield isolated colonies in areas D and E. (b) Poor streaking does not provide separation of colonies.

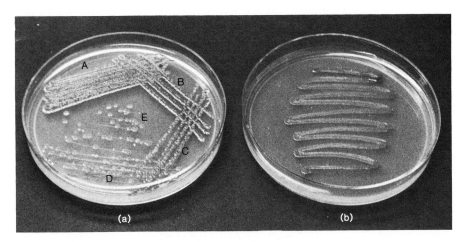

2. Describe each different type of colony you can distinguish.

3. Make a Gram stain of one isolated colony of each type present. Also prepare a Gram stain of the growth in the area where the initial inoculum was placed. (Note: when a stain is to be made of colonies on an agar medium, place a loopful of sterile water or saline on the slide first and then emulsify the picked growth in this drop. Allow to air dry, heat-fix the slide, and stain.)
4. Record your observations in the table provided.

Single Colony	Colony Morphology	Pigment	Gram Reaction	Microscopic Morphology
Serratia marcescens				
Escherichia coli				
Staphylococcus epidermidis				
Area of initial inoculum				

Note: Keep *the nutrient agar plate. You will work with it again in the next exercise.*

B. Examination of Mouth Culture on Blood Agar Plate

1. How many different types of colonies can you find on the blood agar plate? _____
   Describe each.

2. Make a Gram stain of each of three different colonies. Record the Gram reaction of each, and indicate its microscopic morphology.

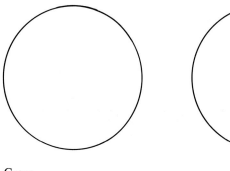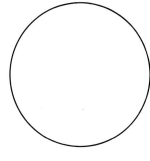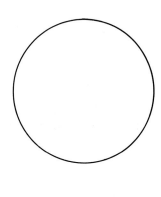

Gram
reaction _____   _____   _____

3. Discard the blood agar plate in a container marked CONTAMINATED.

Questions

1. When an agar plate is inoculated, why is the loop flamed after the initial inoculum is put on?

2. Define a *mixed culture.*

3. Define a *bacterial colony.* List four characteristics by which bacterial colonies may be distinguished.

Basic Techniques of Microbiology

4. Why should a petri dish not be left open for any extended period?

5. Why is the streaking method you used to inoculate your plates called a *streak dilution* technique?

6. Why is it necessary to isolate individual colonies from a mixed growth?

7. Why was a blood agar, rather than a nutrient agar, plate used for the culture from your mouth?

8. Are the large numbers of microorganisms found in the mouth cause for concern? Explain.

9. How do microorganisms find their way into the mouth?

EXERCISE 10 Pour-Plate and Subculture Techniques

Reference: Morello, Mizer, Wilson, and Granato, Microbiology in Patient Care, 5th edition, 1994. Chapter 4.

An alternative method for using agar plates to obtain isolated colonies, other than streaking their surfaces, is to prepare a "pour plate." In this case, an aliquot of the specimen to be cultured is placed in the bottom of an empty, sterile petri dish and melted, then cooled agar is poured over it. Immediately before the agar cools, the plate is gently rocked to disperse the inoculum. When the agar has solidified and the plate is incubated, any bacteria present in the specimen will grow wherever they have been localized, within the agar layer as well as on its surface. Their colonies will be isolated and can be removed from subsurface positions by inserting the inoculating loop or a straight wire into the depth of the agar. It should be noted that the inoculum must be a liquid specimen or culture. If it is not, it must be suspended in sterile fluid before being placed in the petri dish.

Another method for preparing a pour plate is to inoculate the specimen or culture directly into the tube of melted, cooled agar. Mix it by rolling it back and forth between the outstretched fingers of both hands, and pour the inoculated agar into a sterile petri dish. These steps must be performed quickly before the agar cools enough to harden.

When primary isolation plates have been properly poured or streaked, individual colonies can be picked up on an inoculating loop or straight wire and inoculated to fresh agar or broth media. These new pure cultures of isolated organisms are called *subcultures*. If they are indeed pure and do not contain mixtures of different species, they can be identified in stepwise procedures as you will see in later exercises.

Purpose	A. To learn the pour-plate technique for obtaining isolated colonies
	B. To obtain isolated colonies from streak-plate cultures and grow them as pure subcultures
Materials	Tubed nutrient agar (10 ml per tube)
	Sterile petri dishes
	Sterile 1-ml pipettes (cotton plugged)
	Mixed broth culture containing *Escherichia coli* and *Staphylococcus epidermidis*
	Nutrient agar plates (prepared in Exercise 8)
	Nutrient agar broth (prepared in Exercise 8)
	Nutrient agar plate cultures streaked in Exercise 9, containing isolated colonies of three bacterial species

Procedures

A. Pour-Plate Technique

1. Place a tube of sterile nutrient agar in a boiling water bath. (A simple water bath can be set up by placing a glass beaker or tin can half filled with water on a tripod over a Bunsen flame. An asbestos mat must be used under glass vessels. The water should be kept at a steady but not rapid boil. Keep the water level at the halfway mark. An electric burner may be used instead.)
2. When the agar is liquefied, remove the tube and allow it to cool to about 50°C.
3. Place an empty sterile petri dish before you, top side up.
4. Remove a sterile 1-ml pipette from its container, keeping your fingers on the plugged mouth end. Pass the distal one-third of the pipette rapidly through your Bunsen flame (don't overheat it).

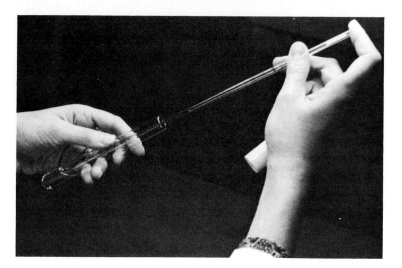

5. Pick up the mixed broth culture in the other hand, remove its closure with the little finger of the hand holding the pipette (*do not touch the latter to anything*), flame the mouth of the open tube, and insert the pipette into the broth.

6. Holding the tube and pipette vertically, poise your index finger over the pipette mouth. Allow the pipette to fill to the level of the broth in the tube and then close off its mouth with your finger (there should be about 0.3 to 0.4 ml of culture in the pipette).

7. Keeping your finger pressed on its top, raise the pipette until the tip is free of the broth and then slowly allow the material in the pipette to run back into the tube until only the last 0.1 ml remains. Now press your finger tightly to close the pipette's mouth and prevent further dripping (fig. 10.1). **Never use your mouth to draw fluid into a pipette.**

8. Before you withdraw the pipette from the tube, touch its tip against the dry inner wall to remove any drop hanging from it.

9. Withdraw the closed pipette, flame the tube, replace its closure, and put the tube down in the rack.

10. Now, with your free hand, remove the top of the petri dish (do not put it down), place the tip of the pipette against the bottom of the dish, release your finger from the mouth, and let 0.1 ml of broth culture run into the plate bottom.

11. Replace the dish top and discard the pipette into a container of disinfectant.

12. Pick up the tube of melted, cool agar, remove its closure, and put it down anywhere. Flame the mouth of the open tube.

13. With your free hand, remove the top of the petri dish (again, do not put it down). Quickly pour the agar into the dish.

14. Replace the petri dish cover (the tube may be set aside for washing). Gently rock the closed dish, or rotate it in circular fashion on the bench top, being careful not to allow the still melted agar to wave up over the edge of the bottom half or onto the cover.

15. Let the agar solidify without further disturbance. When it is quite firm (about 30 minutes), invert the plate and place it in the 35°C incubator.

B. Subculture Technique (Picking Isolated Colonies for Pure Culture)

1. Look again at figure 2.6 in Exercise 2. This figure illustrates the correct method of picking a single colony from the surface of a streaked plate.
2. Now open the nutrient agar plate you streaked in Exercise 9 from a mixed broth culture containing three organisms. Hold the exposed agar surface in good light so that you can see all facets of individual isolated colonies.
3. With your flamed, cooled loop held steady in your other hand, bring the loop edge down against the top surface of one isolated colony you have selected for pure subculture. Withdraw the charged loop (don't touch it to anything!) and close the streaked plate.
4. Inoculate a fresh, sterile nutrient broth by gently rubbing the charged loop against the inner wall of the tube, just beneath the fluid surface. When you bring the loop out of the tube, be sure it holds some of the broth.
5. Now use the loop to inoculate a fresh nutrient agar plate. Rub the inoculum onto a small area near the edge, flame the loop, and then go back and complete the streaking of the plate by the "streak dilution" technique (review fig. 9.1).
6. Inoculate two more agar plates, each with a different type of colony picked from your previous plate culture.
7. Incubate your new plate cultures (inverted) and broth cultures at 35°C.

Results

A. Examination of Pour Plate

Diagram the distribution of colonies you can see in your pour-plate culture (surface and subsurface locations, separation). Indicate any colonial distinctions you can recognize.

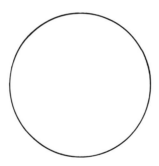

B. Examination of Streaked Plate Subcultures

1. Examine your streaked nutrient agar plate subcultures and determine whether you have obtained pure cultures. In the following table, indicate the size, shape, and pigmentation of colonies on each plate. Make Gram stains of colonies on each subculture plate and record Gram reactions in the table.

Organism	Colony Size (mm, diameter)	Colony Shape	Pigment Color	Gram Reaction	Microscopic Morphology
Escherichia coli					
Serratia marcescens					
Staphylococcus epidermidis					

2. Examine your nutrient broth subcultures. Make Gram stains to determine whether they are pure. Describe your microscopic observations of each broth subculture on the following lines:

_____

_____

_____

3. Are the organisms recovered in your plate and broth cultures the same as those you originally recorded in Exercise 9?

_____

_____

If not, specify the differences: _____

_____

Questions

1. Discuss the relative convenience of pour- and streak-plate techniques in culturing clinical specimens.

2. Why are plate cultures incubated in the inverted position?

3. How do you decide which colonies should be picked from a plate culture of a mixed flora?

4. Why is it necessary to make pure subcultures of organisms grown from clinical specimens?

5. How can you determine whether a culture, or subculture, is pure?

6. What kinds of clinical specimens may yield a mixed flora in bacterial cultures?

7. When more than one colony type appears in a pure culture, what are the most likely sources of the extraneous organisms?

EXERCISE 11 Culturing Microorganisms from the Environment

Reference: Morello, Mizer, Wilson, and Granato, Microbiology in Patient Care, *5th edition, 1994. Chapters 3, 5 (see also 8, 9).*

Microorganisms are found throughout the environment: in the air and water; on the surface of objects, clothes, tables, floors; in soil and dust; and on the surface tissues of our own bodies (skin and mucous membranes).

These ubiquitous microorganisms ordinarily are of no concern to healthy humans, provided we maintain standards of good hygiene in our daily living. In hospitals, however, where susceptible patients must be protected from hospital-acquired (*nosocomial*) infections, the concentration and distribution of microorganisms in the environment are a matter of great importance. Frequent monitoring of the environment is one of the responsibilities of the hospital epidemiologist, who may be a microbiologist, nurse, or physician.

Purpose	To take cultures from selected areas of the environment, in order to identify sources of contaminating microorganisms
Materials	Nutrient broth Nutrient agar plates Sterile swabs

Procedures

1. Place a swab in a nutrient broth to moisten it. As you withdraw the swab, press it against the inner wall of the tube to drain off excess fluid.
2. Take a culture of the floor with this swab by rubbing and rotating it over an area approximately 10 cm square.
3. Inoculate an agar plate with the swab by rotating it over a small area near one edge. Discard the swab and use your wire loop to streak out the plate by the streak dilution technique.
4. Moisten another swab in broth and take a culture of the sink faucet in the area around the aerator or strainer. Inoculate and streak another agar plate as in step 3.
5. Take a fresh agar plate and touch separate areas of the agar surface with each fingertip of your right hand.
6. Take an agar plate into the lavatory. Place it on a shelf or the basin, remove the top, and leave the agar exposed for 30 minutes. Close, invert, and incubate the plate at 35°C.
7. Look around the laboratory for any area where dust has accumulated (window ledges, open shelves, hard-to-clean areas). Take a culture of dust with a moist swab, inoculate, and streak an agar plate.
8. Take a culture (with a moist swab) of a 5-cm square area on the front of your laboratory coat. Inoculate and streak a plate.
9. Run a moist swab through your hair. Inoculate and streak a plate.
10. Incubate all plates, inverted, at 35°C.

Results

Examine all plates and record your observations in the following table.

Source of Specimen	Approximate Number of Colonies	Numbers of Different Colony Types	Gram-Stain Reaction 2 Colony Types	Microscopic Morphology 2 Colony Types

Questions

1. Did you find more gram-positive or gram-negative organisms:

   On the surface of your fingers? _____

   In dust? _____

   In the faucet? _____

   On your clothes? _____

   Can you account for any differences? _____

2. Did you find any endospore-forming bacteria in your cultures? If so, which cultures?

3. In what areas of a hospital must the numbers of microorganisms in the environment be strictly reduced to the minimum?

4. Why do microbiologists wear laboratory coats? Did you confirm that this is necessary?

5. Why is it necessary to wear clean, protective clothing when caring for a patient?

6. Why should hair be kept clean and controlled when caring for patients?

7. How can the numbers of microorganisms in the environment be controlled?

8. When and why is hand washing important in patient care?

9. How can those who care for patients avoid spreading microorganisms among them?

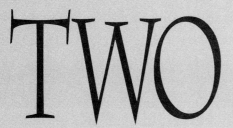
Destruction of Microorganisms

Understanding how microorganisms can be destroyed is of utmost importance in patient-care situations, as well as in the laboratory. Many physical and chemical agents have antimicrobial activity; that is, they act against (anti-) microbes. Among the numerous physical agents that are antimicrobial, heat is the most effective and reliable. It is also more efficient than most antimicrobial chemical agents because it can destroy microbes more rapidly under the right conditions. Chemical agents that are useful for destroying pathogenic microorganisms in the environment, where the application of heat is impractical, are referred to collectively as *disinfectants.* The principles of heat sterilization and chemical disinfection are continuously applied to control infection and are an integral part of patient care. They are also essential to laboratory safety and must be understood before we proceed to the study of pathogenic microorganisms, with which diagnostic microbiology is concerned.

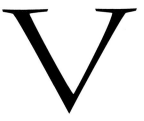

SECTION V

Physical Antimicrobial Agents

We can be assured of complete destruction of *all* forms of microbial life only by using *sterilizing* techniques (the term *sterilization* is an absolute one; it means total, irreversible destruction of living cells). A number of *physical* environmental agents exert a stress on microorganisms and may kill them (ultraviolet or ionizing radiations, ultrasonic waves, or total dryness), but they cannot be relied upon to destroy large concentrations of microorganisms in a laboratory culture or a clinical specimen. Even small numbers of microorganisms may not be totally destroyed if they are evenly distributed in (and protected by) the fabrics contained in a clean surgical pack, which is exposed to ultraviolet rays or dried.

Ultraviolet light does not penetrate most substances, including fabrics, and therefore is used primarily to inactivate microorganisms located on surfaces. In microbiology laboratories, ultraviolet lamps are used inside of biological safety cabinets to decontaminate their surfaces, usually at the end of the day.

Of all the physical agents that exert antimicrobial effects, *heat* is the most effective. It is an excellent sterilizing agent when applied in appropriate intensity for an adequate period of time, because it effectively stops cellular activities. Depending on whether it is moist or dry, heat can coagulate cellular proteins (think of a boiled egg) or oxidize cell components (think of a burned finger or a flaming piece of paper). Heat is also nonselective in its effects on microorganisms (or other living cells), but we must bear in mind that this advantage is offset by its undiscriminating capacity to destroy all materials, viable or not.

In the following exercises, we shall see some examples of the application of moist and dry heat to accomplish sterilization.

EXERCISE 12 Moist and Dry Heat

Reference: Morello, Mizer, Wilson, and Granato, Microbiology in Patient Care, *5th edition, 1994.*
Chapters 2, 9.

In order to sterilize a given set of materials, the appropriate conditions of heat and moisture must be used. Moist heat coagulates microbial proteins (including protein enzymes), inactivating them irreversibly. In the dry state, protein structures are more stable; therefore, the temperature of dry heat must be raised much higher and maintained longer than that of moist heat. For example, in a dry oven, 1 to 2 hours at 160 to 170°C is required; however, with steam under pressure (the autoclave, see Exercise 13), only 15 minutes at 121°C may be needed. The choice of heat sterilization methods then becomes a matter of judging the heat sensitivity of materials to be sterilized.

EXPERIMENT 12.1 Moist Heat

It is possible to quantitate the response of microorganisms to heat by measuring the time required to kill them at different temperatures. The lowest temperature required to sterilize a standardized pure culture (of bacteria) within a given time (usually 10 minutes) can be called the *thermal death point* of that species, and, conversely, the time required to sterilize the culture at a stated temperature can be established as the *thermal death time.*

Purpose	To demonstrate destruction of microorganisms by moist heat applied under controlled conditions of time and temperature
Materials	Tubed nutrient broths (5-ml aliquots) Nutrient agar plates Sterile 1.0-ml pipettes 24-hour broth culture of *Staphylococcus epidermidis* Six-day-old broth culture of *Bacillus subtilis*

Procedures

1. Set up a beaker water bath and heat to boiling.
2. Streak a loopful of the *S. epidermidis* culture onto a nutrient agar plate. Label the plate with the name of the organism and the word *Control.*
3. Repeat procedure 2 with the culture of *B. subtilis.*
4. Place both "control" plates in the 35°C incubator for 24 hours.
5. Take a pair of broth tubes and inoculate each, respectively, with 0.1 ml of *S. epidermidis* and *B. subtilis.* Place these tubes in the boiling water bath. Note the time.
6. Leave the pair of broth cultures in boiling water for 5 minutes. Remove the tubes and cool them quickly under running cold tap water. Streak a loopful of each boiled culture onto a plate of nutrient agar. Label each tube with the name of the organism and the time boiled. (Other members of the class will make identical cultures, but boil them for 10, 15, and 30 minutes, respectively.)
7. Incubate subcultures from boiled tubes at 35°C for 24 hours.

Results

1. Read all plates for growth (+) or no growth (−). Record your own results and those of your neighbors:

Culture	Minutes Boiled				Control
	5	10	15	30	
S. epidermidis					
B. subtilis					

2. State your interpretation of these results for each organism:

   S. epidermidis:

   B. subtilis:

EXPERIMENT 12.2   Dry Heat

In this experiment, egg white (the protein, albumin) is used to simulate microbial enzyme protein. The speed of the damaging reaction (coagulation) of moist and dry heat on protein will be observed.

Purpose	To compare the effects of moist and dry heat
Materials	Tubed distilled water (0.5-ml aliquots) Sterile 1.0-ml pipettes Clean tubes Dry-heat oven Egg white (albumin, a protein)

Procedures

1. Set up a beaker water bath and heat to boiling.
2. Set the dry-heat oven for 100°C.
3. Using a pipette, measure 0.5 ml of egg white into 0.5 ml of distilled water.
4. Place the tube into the boiling water bath and *immediately* begin timing. Observe until the egg white has coagulated, then record the elapsed time.
5. Using a pipette, measure 1.0 ml of egg white into a clean tube.
6. Place the tube into the dry-heat oven and *immediately* begin timing. Observe until the egg white has coagulated, then record the elapsed time.

Results

1. Elapsed time for protein coagulation in moist heat (boiling): _____

   Elapsed time for protein coagulation in dry heat (baking): _____

2. State your interpretation of the effect of moisture on protein denaturation: _____

   _____

EXPERIMENT **12.3**   **Incineration**

Purpose	To learn the effect of flaming with dry heat
Materials	Nutrient agar plates 24-hour broth culture of *Staphylococcus epidermidis* Six-day-old culture of *Bacillus subtilis*

Procedures

1. With your marking pencil, section an agar plate into two parts.
2. Streak the *S. epidermidis* culture on one-half of the plate. Label this section *Control.*
3. Flame the loop, take another loopful of *S. epidermidis* culture, and flame the loop again. When the loop is cool, use it to streak the second half of the plate. Label this section *Flamed.*
4. Repeat procedures 1 to 3 with the *B. subtilis* culture.
5. Incubate the plates at 35°C for 24 hours.

Results

Read for growth (+) or no growth (−) and record.

Organism	Control	Incineration
S. epidermidis		
B. subtilis		

Questions

1. How are microorganisms destroyed by moist heat? By dry heat?

2. Are some microorganisms more resistant to heat than others? Why?

3. Is moist heat more effective than dry heat? Why?

4. Why does dry heat require higher temperatures for longer time periods to sterilize than does moist heat?

5. What is the relationship of time to temperature in heat sterilization? Explain.

6. Would you recommend boiling or baking to sterilize a soiled surgical instrument? Why?

7. What kinds of clean hospital materials would you sterilize by baking? Why?

8. Name some hospital materials that could be sterilized by flaming without harming them.

Destruction of Microorganisms

EXERCISE 13 The Autoclave

Reference: Morello, Mizer, Wilson, and Granato, Microbiology in Patient Care, *5th edition, 1994. Chapter 9.*

The autoclave is a steam-pressure sterilizer. Steam is the vapor given off by water when it boils at 100°C. If steam is trapped and compressed, its temperature rises as the pressure on it increases. As pressure is exerted on a vapor or gas to keep it enclosed within a certain area, the energy of the gaseous molecules is concentrated and exerts equal pressure against the opposing force. The energy of pressurized gas generates heat as well as force. Thus, the temperature of steam produced at 100°C rises sharply above this level if the steam is trapped within a chamber that permits it to accumulate but not to escape. A kitchen pressure cooker illustrates this principle because it is, indeed, an "autoclave." When a pressure cooker containing a little water is placed over a hot burner, the water soon comes to a boil. If the lid of the cooker is then clamped down tightly while heating continues, steam continues to be generated but, having nowhere to go, creates pressure as its temperature climbs steeply. This device may be used in the kitchen to speed cooking of food, because pressurized steam and its high temperature (120 to 125°C) penetrates raw meats and vegetables much more quickly than does boiling water or its dissipating steam. In the process, any microorganisms that may also be present are similarly penetrated by the hot pressurized steam and destroyed.

Essentially, an autoclave is a large, heavy-walled chamber with a steam inlet and an air outlet (fig. 13.1). It can be sealed to force steam accumulation. Steam (being lighter but hotter than air) is admitted through an inlet pipe in the upper part of the rear wall. As it rushes in, it pushes the cool air in the chamber forward and down through an air discharge line in the floor of the chamber at its front. When all the cool air has been pushed down the line, it is followed by hot steam, the temperature of which triggers a thermostatic valve placed in the discharge pipe. The valve closes off the line and now, as steam continues to enter the sealed chamber, pressure and temperature begin to build up quickly. The barometric pressure of normal atmosphere is about 15 lb to the square inch. Within an autoclave, steam pressure can build to 15 to 30 lb per square inch *above* atmospheric pressure, bringing the temperature up with it to 121 to 123°C. Steam is wet and penetrative to begin with, even at 100°C (the boiling point of water). When raised to a high temperature and driven by pressure, it penetrates thick substances that would be only superficially bathed by steam at atmospheric pressure. Under autoclave conditions, pressurized steam kills bacterial endospores, vegetative bacilli, and other microbial forms quickly and effectively at temperatures much lower and less destructive to materials than are required in a dry-heat oven (160 to 170°C).

Temperature and *time* are the two essential factors in heat sterilization. In the autoclave (steam-pressure sterilizer), it is the intensity of *steam temperature* that sterilizes (pressure only provides the means of creating this intensity), when it is given *time* measured according to the nature of the load in the chamber. In the dry-heat oven, the temperature of the hot air (which is not very penetrative) also sterilizes, but only after enough time has been allowed to heat the oven load and oxidize vital components of microorganisms without damaging materials. Table 13.1 illustrates the influence of pressure on the temperature of steam and, in turn, the influence of temperature on the time required to kill heat-resistant bacterial endospores. Compare these figures with those required for an average oven load—160°C for two hours, 170°C for one hour—and you will see the efficiency of steam-pressure sterilization. Timing should not begin in either oven or autoclave sterilization until the interior chamber has reached sterilizing temperature.

The nature of the load in a heating sterilizing chamber greatly influences the time required to sterilize every item within the load. Steam *penetration* of thick, bulky, porous articles, such as operating room linen packs, takes much longer than does steam *condensation* on the surfaces of metal surgical instruments or laboratory glassware (quickly raised to sterilizing temperatures). The packaging of individual items (wrapped, plugged, or basketed) also influences heat penetration, as does the arrangement of the total load in either an autoclave or an oven. In the autoclave, steam must be able to penetrate every surface of every item. In the oven, hot air must circulate freely around each piece in the load to bring it to sterilizing temperature. When sterilizing empty vessels in a steam-pressure sterilizer, for example, it is

Figure 13.1 The autoclave. From Adrian N. C. Delaat, *Microbiology for the Allied Health Professionals*, 2d ed. Copyright 1979 Lea & Febiger, Philadelphia, Pennsylvania. Reprinted by permission.

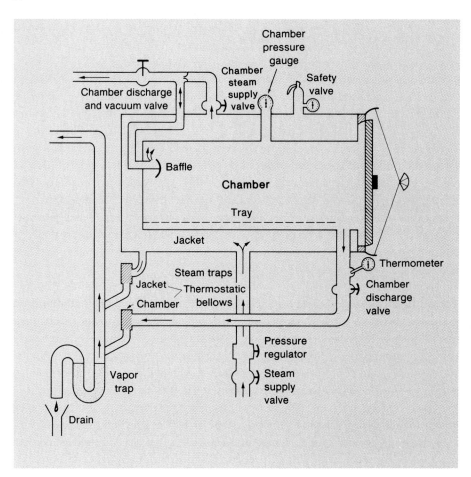

Table 13.1 Pressure-Temperature-Time Relationships in Steam-Pressure Sterilization

Steam Pressure, Pounds per Square Inch (Above Atmospheric Pressure)	Temperature		Time (Minutes Required to Kill Exposed Heat-Resistant Endospores)
	Centigrade	Fahrenheit	
0	100°	212°	—
10	115.5°	240°	15–60
15	121.5°	250°	12–15
20	126.5°	260°	5–12
30	134°	270°	3–5

Destruction of Microorganisms

Figure 13.2 Ampules of *B. stearothermophilus* are used to ensure that sterilization is accomplished in the autoclave. Becton Dickinson Microbiology Systems, Cockeysville, MD.

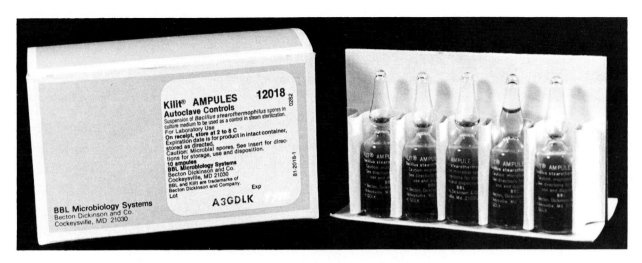

important to consider that they contain cool air. Air is cooler and heavier than steam and cannot be permeated by it; therefore, microorganisms lingering within air pockets existing in or among items placed in an autoclave may survive steam exposure. For this reason, empty vessels (test tubes, syringes, beakers, flasks) should be laid on their sides so that the air they contain can run out and downward and be replaced by steam. Similarly, packaged materials should be positioned so that air pockets are not created among or between them.

Under routine conditions, properly controlled, steam-pressure sterilization can be accomplished under the following conditions of pressure, time, and temperature:

15 to 20 lb of steam pressure
121 to 125°C (250 to 256°F) steam temperature
15 to 45 minutes, depending on the nature of the load

Bacteriologic controls of autoclave efficiency are essential at frequent intervals to ensure that sterilization is being accomplished with each run of the steam-pressure sterilizer. Preparations of heat-resistant bacterial endospores are commercially available for this purpose. Such preparations contain viable endospores dried on paper strips or suspended in nutrient broth within a sealed ampule (fig. 13.2). When appropriately placed within an autoclave load, endospore controls can reveal whether the autoclave is operating efficiently, mechanically; individual item packaging is correct; and load arrangement permits sterilization of every item within the load.

The endospores of a bacterial species called *Bacillus stearothermophilus* provide a highly critical test of autoclave procedures, because they are extremely resistant to the effects of moist or dry heat. As their name implies, they are heat (*thermo-*) -loving (*-philus*), but this also means that they require a higher incubation temperature than is optimal for most bacteria. The vegetative cells of *B. stearothermophilus* grow best at *56°C* rather than at the 35°C temperature that is optimal for most pathogenic microorganisms. When dried on paper strips, these endospores provide a good test of oven sterilization techniques. When suspended in broth in sealed ampules, they are very useful for testing autoclave performance.

B. stearothermophilus endospores on *paper strips* are packaged within paper envelopes that are placed within a load before heat sterilization. After sterilization, they are removed from their envelopes (aseptically), placed in appropriate nutrient broth, incubated at 56°C, and observed for evidence that they did or did not survive the sterilizing technique. *Sealed ampules* containing endospore suspensions are placed in an autoclave load (they cannot be used to test oven sterilization because they contain liquid), removed, and simply placed, without being opened, in an appropriate incubator (water bath or incubator at 56°C). Within a sealed ampule, endospores have been suspended in a nutrient broth also containing a pH-sensitive dye indicator. If endospores survive autoclaving and germinate again under incubation, vegetative bacilli begin to multiply in the broth. In the process, they use its nutrients, producing acid end products that cause the indicator to change color. They also produce turbidity in the medium.

When strips or ampules are used to test heat-sterilization technique, *unheated* strip or ampule controls must be incubated also to prove that the endospores were viable to begin with. At the completion of the incubation time, evidence of growth should be observed for the *control* but not the heated endospore preparations. If the heated test strips or ampules do not show growth by 24 to 48 hours, incubation should be continued for up to 7 days. The test then may be reported as negative, and the sterilization technique is assumed to have been effective. Patient-care materials included in the sterilized load are now safe to use. If, however, the endospores in the control preparation have not germinated, the test is considered unreliable, and the sterilized material cannot be assumed to be free of contaminating microorganisms. The sterilization procedure should be repeated with a new lot of strips or ampules.

Ampules containing liquid endospore suspensions must be kept refrigerated before use, because warm storage temperatures may permit endospore germination that could be wrongly interpreted. Dried endospore strips may be stored at room temperature because dry endospores are not likely to germinate.

In this exercise, you will have an opportunity to see the sterilizing effects of an autoclave.

Purpose	To illustrate the use and control of an autoclave
Materials	Commercially prepared strips or ampules containing *Bacillus stearothermophilus* endospores*
	Nutrient broth (if strips are used)
	Forceps (if strips are used)
	1.0-ml sterile pipettes
	56°C water bath or incubator
	Phenol red glucose broth tubes
	Six-day-old broth culture of *Bacillus subtilis*

*Some commercially available paper strips (American Sterilizer Company, "Spordex") contain two types of endospores in combination: those of *B. stearothermophilus* and also *B. subtilis*. The latter are less heat resistant than endospores of *B. stearothermophilus* and do not require a high incubation temperature to germinate (35 to 37°C is satisfactory for incubation of *B. subtilis*). These combination strips can therefore be used in either a gas sterilizer, an autoclave, or an oven. In a gas sterilizer, the relatively low temperature will destroy *B. subtilis* endospores but not those of *B. stearothermophilus*. Strips used for this purpose may then be incubated at 35°C to test for the survival of *B. subtilis* (the thermophile will not grow), while strips placed in an autoclave or oven load are incubated at 56°C to test for growth of *B. stearothermophilus* (the mesophile will not grow).

Procedures

1. The instructor will discuss and demonstrate the operation of the autoclave.
2. Inoculate a tube of phenol red glucose broth with 0.1 ml of the *B. subtilis* culture (*finger* the pipette). Label it *Unheated* and place it in the incubator at 35°C for 24 hours.
3. Submit the culture of *B. subtilis* for autoclaving at 15 lb, 121°C, for 15 minutes. Afterward, inoculate a tube of phenol red glucose broth with 0.1 ml of the autoclaved culture. Label it *Autoclaved.* Incubate the glucose broth at 35°C for 24 hours.

Destruction of Microorganisms

4. The instructor will demonstrate the use of endospore controls. An unheated *B. stearothermophilus* endospore preparation will be placed in a 56°C water bath or incubator. Another will be placed in the autoclave with your subculture of *B. subtilis* and then incubated.
   a. If strips are used, the paper envelope of one will be torn open, and the strip will be removed with a flamed forceps and placed in nutrient broth incubated at 56°C. Another will be placed in the autoclave (in its envelope) and heated and then removed and placed in broth.
   b. If ampules are used, one will be placed (unheated, unopened) in the 56°C water bath or incubator. Another will be autoclaved and then incubated without opening.
5. After at least 24 hours of incubation of all cultures, read and examine them for evidence of growth (+) or no growth (−).

Results

1. Record culture results in the following table.

Test Organism	Autoclave				Appearance of Incubated Controls or Glucose Broth Cultures		
	Time	Temp.	Pressure	Incubation Temperature	Color	Turbidity	Growth (+ or −)
B. stearothermophilus Unheated control	x	x	x				
Autoclaved control							
B. subtilis Unheated culture	x	x	x				
Autoclaved culture							

2. State your interpretation of these results:

3. State the method used for timing the autoclave in your experiment:

Questions

1. Define the principles of sterilization with an autoclave and with a dry-heat oven.

2. What pressure, temperature, and time are used in routine autoclaving?

3. What factors determine the time period necessary for steam-pressure sterilization? Dry-heat oven sterilization?

4. Why is it necessary to use bacteriologic controls to monitor heat-sterilization techniques?

5. When running an endospore control of autoclaving technique, why is one endospore preparation incubated without heating?

6. Would a culture of *E. coli* make a good bacteriologic control of heat-sterilization techniques? Why?

7. What characteristics of *B. stearothermophilus* make it valuable for use as a control organism for heat-sterilization techniques? Explain.

8. What factors determine the choice of a paper strip containing bacterial endospores or a sealed ampule containing an endospore suspension for testing heat-sterilization equipment?

9. Would you choose a dry-heat oven, an autoclave, or incineration to heat sterilize the following items? State why.

   Soiled dressings from a surgical wound: _____

   _____

   Surgical instruments: _____

   _____

   Clean laboratory glassware: _____

   _____

   Clean syringes: _____

   _____

10. Why should the results of endospore control tests be known before heat-sterilized materials are used for patient care?

SECTION VI

Chemical Antimicrobial Agents

A wide variety of chemical agents display antimicrobial activity to some degree. In considering their application to patient care, we may separate them into two general classes: (1) those that are useful for destroying pathogenic microorganisms in the environment (*disinfectants*) or on skin (*antiseptics*), and (2) those that may be administered to patients for treatment of infectious diseases (*antimicrobial agents*).

Many antimicrobial substances are too toxic to be used for patient therapy but are valuable as environmental disinfectants. These must be chosen carefully for the job to be done, because a given disinfectant usually does not kill all microbial pathogens. Each agent has a limited chemical mode of action, and microorganisms exposed to it may vary widely in their responses. Some microbes or their forms may succumb to its effects (such as vegetative bacterial cells) whereas others may not (such as bacterial endospores). In the experiments of Exercise 14, we shall study some of the many factors that influence the disinfection process.

Antimicrobial agents are substances that are naturally produced by a variety of microorganisms (primarily fungi and bacteria), or have been synthesized in the laboratory, or a combination of both. For example, scientists in pharmaceutical companies have made many chemical modifications of the penicillin molecule (a product of the fungus *Penicillium notatum*) to broaden its spectrum of activity. In strict use, *antibiotic* refers only to those antimicrobial substances produced by microorganisms, but the term is often used interchangeably with *antimicrobial agent.* Antimicrobial agents have inhibitory or lethal effects on many pathogenic organisms (especially bacteria) that cause infectious diseases. In purified form, they are administered to patients for their antimicrobial effects within the body. In general, each agent has special activity against one or more types of microorganisms (gram-positive bacteria, gram-negative bacteria, fungi, and recently, some viruses).

Like disinfectants, antimicrobial agents have specific chemical modes of action, but the range of activity of antimicrobial agents is narrower. Therefore, as we shall learn in Exercise 15, the diagnostic microbiology laboratory tests the antimicrobial susceptibility of pathogenic bacteria so as to provide the physician with valuable information about the most clinically useful antimicrobial agent to treat a patient's infection specifically. At present, reliable tests for determining fungal and viral susceptibility to antimicrobial agents are not generally available. In addition to the isolation and identification of pathogenic microorganisms that we shall study in sections of Part 3, antimicrobial susceptibility testing is one of the most important functions of the diagnostic microbiology laboratory.

EXERCISE 14 Disinfectants

Reference: Morello, Mizer, Wilson, and Granato, Microbiology in Patient Care, *5th edition, 1994.*
Chapter 9.

Disinfection is defined as the destruction of *pathogenic* microorganisms (not necessarily *all* microbial forms). It is a process involving chemical interactions between a toxic antimicrobial substance and enzymes or other constituents of microbial cells. A disinfectant must kill pathogens while it is in contact with them, so that they cannot grow again when it is removed. In this case it is said to be *cidal* (lethal), and it is described, according to the type of organism it kills, as bactericidal, virucidal, sporicidal, or simply germicidal. If the antimicrobial substance merely inhibits the organisms while it is in contact with them, they may be able to multiply again when it is removed. In this case, the agent is said to have *static* activity (it *arrests* growth) and may be described as bacteriostatic, fungistatic, or virustatic, as the case may be. According to its definition, a chemical disinfectant should produce irreversible changes that are lethal to cells.

Microorganisms of different groups are not uniformly susceptible to chemical disinfection. Tubercle bacilli are more resistant than most other vegetative bacteria because of their waxy cell walls, but of all microbial forms, bacterial endospores display the greatest resistance to both chemical and physical disinfecting agents. Fungal spores are also somewhat resistant, although yeasts and hyphae (nonsporing fungal structures), like bacteria, succumb quickly to active disinfectants. Many bactericidal disinfectants also kill viruses, but the viral agents of hepatitis are very resistant.

Since microorganisms differ in their response to chemical antimicrobial agents, the choice of disinfectant for a particular purpose is guided in part by the type of microbe present in the contaminated material. Disinfectants that effectively kill vegetative bacteria may not destroy bacterial endospores, fungal spores, tubercle bacilli, or some viruses. Other practical factors to consider when choosing a disinfectant include the exposure time and germicide concentration required to kill microorganisms, the temperature and pH for its optimal activity, the concentration of microorganisms present, and the toxicity of the agent for skin or its effect on materials to be disinfected.

Purpose	To study the activity of some disinfectants and to learn the importance of time, germicidal concentration, and microbial species in disinfection
Materials	Nutrient agar plates Sterile, empty tubes Sterile 10-ml pipettes (cotton plugged) Sterile 1.0-ml pipettes (cotton plugged) Bulb or other aspiration device for pipette 1.0% phenol, 2.0% phenol Absolute alcohol, 70% alcohol 3% hydrogen peroxide 1% Lysol, 5% Lysol Iodophor (Betadine) Antiseptic mouthwash 24-hour nutrient broth culture of *Escherichia coli* Three- to six-day-old broth culture of *Bacillus subtilis*

Procedures

1. Select one of the chemical agents provided. Pipette 5.0 ml of the solution into a sterile test tube.
2. To the 5 ml of disinfectant, add 0.5 ml of the *E. coli* culture. Gently shake the tube to distribute the organisms uniformly. Note the time.

3. Divide a nutrient agar plate into four sections with a marking pen or pencil. At intervals of 2, 5, 10, and 15 minutes, transfer one loopful of the disinfectant-culture mixture to a section of the nutrient agar plate. Label each plate with the name of the organism, the disinfectant, and its concentration (for example, *E. coli,* 1% phenol). Label each section of the plate with the time of exposure (for example, 2 minutes, 5 minutes, etc.).
4. Using the same concentration of the same disinfectant, repeat procedures 1 to 3 with the culture of *B. subtilis.*
5. Inoculate one-half of a nutrient agar plate directly from the *E. coli* culture and the other half from the *B. subtilis* culture. Label each half with the name of the organism and the word *Control.*
6. Incubate all tubes at 35°C for 48 hours.

Results

1. Observe all plate sections for growth (+) or absence of growth (−). Complete the following table by recording your own and your neighbors' results with each disinfectant:

Disinfectant	Concentration	Organism	Time of Exposure (Min)				Control
			2	5	10	15	
Phenol	1%	E. coli					
		B. subtilis					
	2%	E. coli					
		B. subtilis					
Alcohol	Absolute	E. coli					
		B. subtilis					
	70%	E. coli					
		B. subtilis					
Hydrogen Peroxide	3%	E. coli					
		B. subtilis					
Lysol	1%	E. coli					
		B. subtilis					
	5%	E. coli					
		B. subtilis					
Iodophor	10%	E. coli					
		B. subtilis					
Mouthwash	*	E. coli					
		B. subtilis					

*Check label of mouthwash bottle; fill in concentration of active ingredient.

Destruction of Microorganisms

2. State your interpretation of these results:

Questions

1. During their laboratory testing, if disinfectants are carried over into microbial cultures, could the results be affected? Explain.

2. Define *disinfection*.

3. What does bactericidal mean? Bacteriostatic? Virucidal? Fungistatic?

4. Why are control cultures necessary in evaluating disinfectants?

5. What factors can influence the activity of a disinfectant?

6. Why do microorganisms differ in their response to disinfectants?

7. What microorganisms are most susceptible to disinfectants?

8. Which microbial forms are most resistant to disinfectants?

9. How can bacteriostatic and bactericidal disinfectants be distinguished?

10. What is an iodophor? What is its value?

11. Did you find the mouthwash you tested to be as effective as the other disinfectants included in this Exercise? Explain any difference you observed.

12. Why are bacterial endospores a problem in the hospital environment?

13. Briefly discuss disinfection in relation to patient care.

EXERCISE 15 Antimicrobial Agents (Antimicrobial Susceptibility Testing)

Reference: Morello, Mizer, Wilson, and Granato, Microbiology in Patient Care, *5th edition, 1994.*
Chapters 4, 9.

An important function of the diagnostic microbiology laboratory is to help the physician select effective antimicrobial agents for specific therapy of infectious diseases. When a clinically significant microorganism is isolated from the patient, it is usually necessary to determine how it responds in vitro to medically useful antimicrobial agents, so that the appropriate drug can be given to the patient. Antimicrobial susceptibility testing of the isolated pathogen indicates which drugs are most likely to inhibit or destroy it in vivo.

EXPERIMENT 15.1 Agar Disk Diffusion Method

The testing method most frequently used is the standardized *filter paper disk agar diffusion* method, also known as the *NCCLS* (National Committee for Clinical Laboratory Standards) or *Bauer-Kirby* method. In this test, a number of small, sterile filter paper disks of uniform size (6 mm) that have each been impregnated with a defined concentration of an antimicrobial agent are placed on the surface of an agar plate previously inoculated with a standard amount of the organism to be tested. The plate is inoculated with uniform, close streaks to assure that the microbial growth will be confluent and evenly distributed across the entire plate surface. Using a disk dispenser or sterile forceps, the disks are placed in even array on the plate, at well-spaced intervals from each other. When the disks are in firm contact with the agar, the antimicrobial agents diffuse into the surrounding medium and come in contact with the multiplying organisms. The plates are incubated at 35°C for 18 to 24 hours.

After incubation, the plates are examined for the presence of zones of inhibition of bacterial growth (clear rings) around the antimicrobial disks (see colorplate 14). If there is no inhibition, growth extends up to the rim of the disks on all sides and the organism is reported as resistant (R) to the antimicrobial agent in that disk. If a zone of inhibition surrounds the disk, the organism is not automatically considered susceptible (S) to the drug being tested. The diameter of the zone must first be measured (in millimeters) and compared for size with values listed in a standard chart (Table 15.1). The size of the zone of inhibition depends on a number of factors, including the rate of diffusion of a given drug in the medium, the degree of susceptibility of the organism to the drug, the number of organisms inoculated on the plate, and their rate of growth. It is essential, therefore, that the test be performed in a fully standardized manner so that the values read from the chart provide an accurate interpretation of susceptibility or resistance. In some instances, the organism cannot be classified as either susceptible or resistant, but is interpreted as being of "intermediate" or "indeterminate" (I) susceptibility to a given drug. If the physician wants to use such a drug to treat the patient, additional tests are usually necessary to assess the susceptibility of the organism more precisely.

A fourth category, used instead of I with some microorganisms and antimicrobial agents, is "moderately susceptible" (MS). The clinical interpretation of this category is that the organisms tested may be inhibited by the antimicrobial agent provided that either (1) higher doses of drug are given to the patient, or (2) the infection is at a body site where the drug is concentrated; for example, the penicillins are excreted from the body by the kidneys and reach higher concentrations in the urinary tract than in the bloodstream or tissues. When either an I or MS interpretation is obtained, the physician may wish to select an alternative antimicrobial agent to which the infecting microorganism is fully susceptible.

Table 15.1   Zone Diameter Interpretive Table

Antimicrobial Agent	Disk Concentration	Diameter of Inhibition Zone (mm)			
		R	I	MS	S
Ampicillin[a]	10 µg	≤13	—	14–16	≥17
Carbenicillin[b]	100 µg	≤13	—	14–16	≥17
Cefoxitin	30 µg	≤14	—	15–17	≥18
Cephalothin	30 µg	≤14	—	15–17	≥18
Clindamycin	2 µg	≤14	15–20	—	≥21
Erythromycin	15 µg	≤13	14–22	—	≥23
Gentamicin	10 µg	≤12	13–14	—	≥15
Methicillin[c]	5 µg	≤ 9	10–13	—	≥14
Penicillin G[c]	10 U	≤28	—	—	≥29
Penicillin G[d]	10 U	≤14	—	≥15	—
Sulfonamides	250 or 300 µg	≤12	—	13–16	≥17
Tetracycline	30 µg	≤14	15–18	—	≥19
Vancomycin	30 µg	≤ 9	10–11	—	≥12

Source: Adapted from *Performance Standards for Antimicrobial Disk Susceptibility Tests*—Fourth Informational Supplement (M100–S4). National Committee for Clinical Laboratory Standards, NCCLS, 1992. The material is constantly being updated, and you should obtain the latest information from NCCLS.

Notes: Zone sizes appropriate only when testing

[a]Gram-negative enteric organisms

[b]*Pseudomonas*

[c]Staphylococci

[d]Enterococci

Purpose	To learn the agar disk diffusion technique for antimicrobial susceptibility testing
Materials	Nutrient agar plates (Mueller-Hinton if available) Tubes of sterile nutrient broth or saline (5 ml each) Antimicrobial disks (various drugs in standard concentrations) Antimicrobial disk dispenser (optional) McFarland No. 0.5 turbidity standard Sterile swabs Forceps Beaker containing 70% alcohol 24-hour plate cultures of *Staphylococcus epidermidis* and *Escherichia coli*

Procedures

1. Touch 4 to 5 colonies of *S. epidermidis* with your flamed and cooled inoculating loop. Emulsify the colonies in 5 ml of sterile broth or saline until the turbidity is approximately equivalent to that of the McFarland No. 0.5 turbidity standard.
2. Dip a swab into the bacterial suspension, express any excess fluid against the side of the tube, and inoculate the surface of an agar plate as follows: first streak the whole surface of the plate closely with the swab; then rotate the plate through a 45° angle and streak the whole surface again; finally rotate the plate another 90° and streak once more. Discard the swab in disinfectant.
3. Repeat procedures 1 and 2 with the *E. coli* broth culture on a second nutrient agar plate.
4. Dip the tips of the forceps in 70% alcohol, flame rapidly, and allow to cool.

5. Pick up an antimicrobial disk with the forceps and place it on the agar surface of one of the inoculated plates. Press the disk gently into full contact with the agar, using the tips of the forceps.
6. Dip the forceps in alcohol, flame, and cool.
7. Repeat procedures 5 and 6 until about eight different disks are in place on one plate, spaced evenly away from each other. (If an antimicrobial disk dispenser is available, all disks may be dispensed on the agar surface simultaneously. Be certain to press them into contact with the agar using the forceps tips.)
8. Place a duplicate of each disk on the other inoculated plate, using the same procedures.
9. Invert the plates and incubate them at 35°C for 18 to 24 hours.

Results

Observe for the presence or absence of growth around each antimicrobial disk on each plate culture. Using a ruler with millimeter markings, measure the diameters of any zones of inhibition and record them in the following chart. If the organism grows right up to the edge of a disk, record a zone diameter of 6 mm (the diameter of the disk).

| Antimicrobial Agent | Concentration | Zone Diameter | | E. coli (S, MS, I, or R) | S. epidermidis (S, MS, I, or R) |
		E. coli	S. epider-midis		

EXPERIMENT 15.2   Broth Dilution Method: Determining Minimum Inhibitory Concentration (MIC)

In certain instances of life-threatening infections such as bacterial endocarditis, or infections caused by highly or multiply resistant organisms, the physician may require a *quantitative* assessment of microorganism susceptibility rather than the qualitative report of S, MS, I, or R. The laboratory then tests the susceptibility of the organism to varying concentrations of one or more appropriate antimicrobial agents. Twofold dilutions of each antimicrobial agent are prepared over a range of concentrations that are achievable in the patient's bloodstream or urine (depending on the infection site) when standard doses of the drug are administered. In some cases, rather than preparing a full series of twofold dilutions, the organism is tested in only two or three antimicrobial concentrations. In this *breakpoint dilution* method, the concentrations tested are chosen carefully to discriminate between susceptible and resistant organisms.

The antimicrobial dilutions may be prepared in a broth medium, or each concentration of antimicrobial agent to be tested can be incorporated into an agar medium. In this *agar dilution method* many organisms (up to 32) can be tested on a single agar plate although several plates, each containing a different antimicrobial concentration, are needed to perform the assay. When only a single organism is tested, the *broth dilution method* is more rapid and economical to perform. Many laboratories now use commercially available microdilution plates. These consist of multiwelled plastic plates prefilled with various dilutions of several antimicrobial agents in broth (see colorplate 15). Using a multipronged device, the microwells are inoculated simultaneously with a standardized suspension of the test organism. Thus the susceptibility of an organism to many antimicrobial agents may be readily tested.

Regardless of the dilution method chosen, the results are interpreted in the same manner. After 18 to 24 hours of incubation at 35°C, the broths or plates are examined for inhibition of bacterial growth. For each antimicrobial agent, the *lowest* concentration that inhibits growth is referred to as the minimum inhibitory concentration or MIC. As with the disk agar diffusion method, in order to obtain accurate information, variables such as inoculum size, phase of organism growth, broth or agar medium used, and antimicrobial agent storage conditions must be rigidly controlled.

Purpose	To learn the broth dilution method for antimicrobial susceptibility testing
Materials	Nutrient broth (Mueller-Hinton if available)
	Sterile tubes
	Broth containing 128 μg of ampicillin per ml
	Sterile 1- and 5-ml pipettes
	Bulb or other aspiration device for pipette
	Tubes of sterile saline (5.0 and 9.9 ml per tube)
	Overnight plate culture of *Escherichia coli*

Procedures

1. Place nine sterile tubes in a rack and label them as follows:

Tube No.:	1	2	3	4	5	6	7	8	9
Label:	64	32	16	8	4	2	1	Growth Control	Sterility Control

2. With a 5-ml pipette add 0.5 ml of sterile broth to *each* tube.
3. Add 0.5 ml of the ampicillin broth to the first tube (fig. 15.1a). Discard the pipette. The concentration of ampicillin in this tube is 64 μg per ml.
4. Take a fresh pipette, introduce it into the first tube (64 μg per ml), mix the contents thoroughly, and transfer 0.5 ml from this tube into the second tube (32 μg per ml). Discard the pipette.
5. With a fresh pipette, mix the contents of the second tube and transfer 0.5 ml to the third tube (16 μg per ml).
6. Continue the dilution process through tube number 7. The eighth and ninth tubes receive no antibiotic.
7. After the contents of the seventh tube are mixed, discard 0.5 ml of broth so that the final volume in all tubes is 0.5 ml.
8. From the plate culture of *E. coli* prepare a suspension of the organism in 5 ml of saline equivalent to a McFarland 0.5 standard (see Exp. 15.1).
9. With a sterile 1-ml pipette, transfer 0.1 ml of the *E. coli* suspension into a tube containing 9.9 ml of saline. Discard the pipette.
10. With a fresh pipette, mix the contents of the tube well. Add 0.1 ml of this organism suspension to the antibiotic-containing broth tubes 1 through 7 and to the growth control tube (fig. 15.1b).
11. Shake the rack gently to mix the tube contents and place the tubes in the incubator for 18 to 24 hours.

Destruction of Microorganisms

Name _____ Class _____ Date _____

Figure 15.1 Broth dilution technique. (a) The ampicillin-containing broth is serially diluted in tubes that have been filled with 0.5 ml of a nutrient broth. The growth and sterility control tubes receive no antibiotic. (b) After the antimicrobial dilutions are completed, 0.1 ml of the appropriately diluted organism suspension, in this case *E. coli*, is added to all except the sterility control tube. The number on each tube is the final concentration of ampicillin in that tube (μg/ml).

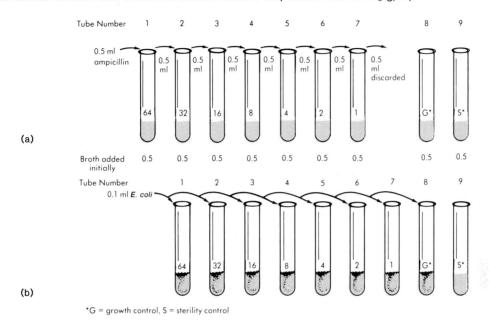

*G = growth control, S = sterility control

Results

Examine each tube for the presence or absence of turbidity. Record the results in the following chart and indicate the MIC of ampicillin for the *E. coli* strain tested.

Antimicrobial Concentration (μg/ml)	64	32	16	8	4	2	1	Growth Control	Sterility Control
Growth (+ or −)									
MIC = _____ μg/ml									

EXPERIMENT **15.3**   **Bacterial Resistance to Antimicrobial Agents**

The activity of antimicrobial agents is usually very specific, affecting primarily essential bacterial cell structures or biochemical processes. For example, penicillin interferes with bacterial cell wall synthesis, gentamicin inhibits protein synthesis, and sulfonamides block folic acid synthesis. During the few decades of widespread antimicrobial agent usage, it has become evident that bacteria have the ability to inactivate or in some way circumvent the activity of almost every known agent. Resistance to antimicrobial agents can result from a mutation in a gene on the bacterial chromosome, or by acquisition from another organism of a plasmid (extrachromosomal DNA) that bears one or more "resistance" genes (R-factor). Acquisition of an R-factor can suddenly render a previously susceptible bacterium resistant to multiple antimicrobial agents. One of the most common mechanisms of bacterial resistance is the production of specific enzymes

Figure 15.2 Penicillin G (shown) and many of its derivatives are inactivated by a beta-lactamase (penicillinase). The enzyme breaks open the beta-lactam ring, which is a common part of the molecular structure of these antimicrobial agents.

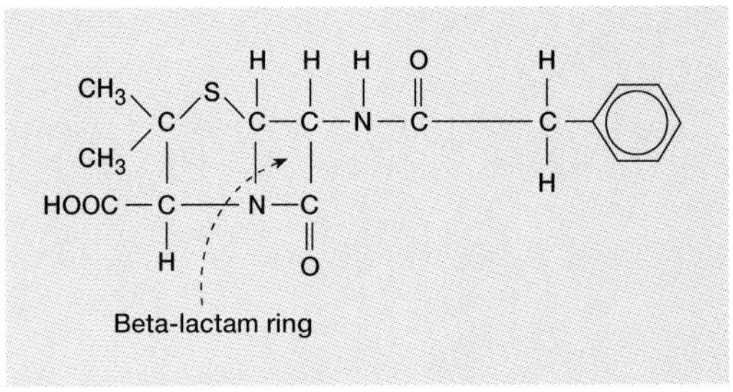

Beta-lactam ring

(see also Exercise 18) that destroy antimicrobial agents before they can affect the bacterium. For example, penicillinase is an enzyme that inactivates penicillin by breaking open a particular structure on the penicillin molecule called a beta-lactam ring (a synonym for penicillinase is beta-lactamase) (fig. 15.2). A gene on a plasmid in the bacterial cell provides instructions for formation of this enzyme. Although carriage of the penicillinase plasmid once appeared to be confined to certain strains of staphylococci and gram-negative bacilli, it is now being found in some strains of bacteria that previously were considered to be universally susceptible to penicillin or its derivatives. These include *Haemophilus influenzae,* a cause of severe infections in children, and *Neisseria gonorrhoeae,* the agent of gonorrhea.

Bacterial enzymes can also be responsible for resistance to antimicrobial agents other than penicillin. Gentamicin and chloramphenicol, for example, may be inactivated by enzymes specific for these drugs, but there are additional mechanisms by which bacteria may resist the action of certain antimicrobial agents. These include alterations in critical bacterial enzymes or proteins such that they can no longer be directly affected by the drug; or changes in the bacterial cell wall or membrane that make the cell less permeable, preventing entrance of the agent.

Routinely, the clinical microbiology laboratory tests for bacterial susceptibility or resistance by the methods described in Experiments 15.1 and 15.2. Alternatively, however, if you are interested only in the response of a given organism to a particular antimicrobial agent (e.g., *Neisseria gonorrhoeae* to penicillin), you can test the organism for its ability to produce a sufficient amount of an enzyme that specifically inactivates that drug. If the organism can be shown to possess the enzyme, it is considered to be resistant to the antimicrobial agent in question. One such test is illustrated in the following experiment, using a penicillin-susceptible organism and one that is resistant to penicillin because it produces penicillinase. The test uses a filter paper disk containing the chromogenic (color-producing) cephalosporin, nitrocefin. Like penicillin, the cephalosporins are degraded by beta-lactamases. When the test disk is inoculated with a penicillinase-producing organism, the yellow nitrocefin is broken down to a red end product.

Purpose	To detect penicillinase production by a test bacterial strain
Materials	Filter paper disks impregnated with nitrocefin for performing the beta-lactamase test
	Sterile water or saline
	Clean glass slides
	Forceps
	Plate culture of a penicillin-resistant *Staphylococcus aureus*
	Plate culture of a penicillin-susceptible *Bacillus subtilis*

Procedures

1. Place two small drops of water or saline on the surface of a clean glass slide.
2. Pick up a beta-lactamase disk with your forceps and place it in contact with one drop of fluid.
3. Repeat this procedure with a second disk, placing it on the second drop of fluid. Do not oversaturate the disks.

4. With your flamed and cooled inoculating loop, pick up a portion of a *B. subtilis* colony and rub it across the surface of the first disk.
5. Rub a portion of a *S. aureus* colony across the surface of the second disk.
6. Observe the areas on the beta-lactamase disks where the organisms were inoculated for up to 30 minutes. A positive result is usually seen within 3 to 4 minutes.

Results

1. A change in the color of the bacterial growth rubbed on the disk from yellow to red is a positive test indicating degradation of nitrocefin.
2. Record your results in the following chart.

Organism	Color on strip after 30 min.	Penicillinase + or −
B. subtilis		
S. aureus		

Questions

1. Define an *antimicrobial agent*.

2. What is meant by antimicrobial resistance? Susceptibility?

3. Why are pure cultures used for antimicrobial susceptibility testing?

4. Would it be acceptable to use a mixed culture for this test? Why?

5. List three factors that can influence the accuracy of the test.

6. If a McFarland 0.5 standard contains 1×10^8 organisms per milliliter, how many bacteria were added to each ampicillin-containing tube in Experiment 15.2?

7. When performing a broth dilution test, why is it necessary to include a growth control tube? A sterility control tube?

8. How can the *minimum bactericidal concentration* of an antimicrobial agent be determined from an MIC assay?

9. Could an organism that is susceptible to an antimicrobial agent in laboratory testing fail to respond to it when that drug is used to treat the patient? Explain.

10. Are antibacterial agents useful in viral infections? Explain.

11. Why is it better to use the word *susceptible* rather than the word *sensitive* in describing an organism's response to a drug? When speaking of the patient, what does the term *drug sensitivity* mean?

12. Describe a mechanism of bacterial resistance to antimicrobial agents.

13. If the laboratory isolates *S. aureus* from five patients on the same day, is it necessary to test the antimicrobial susceptibility of each isolate? Why?

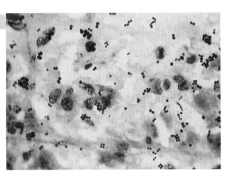

Plate 1 Staphylococci (*Staphylococcus aureus*) in a Gram-stained smear from an abscess. The organisms appear as purple (gram-positive) spheres, primarily in grapelike clusters. Some cells also occur singly or in short chains. The large pink cells are polymorphonuclear neutrophils. Courtesy Dr. E. J. Bottone.

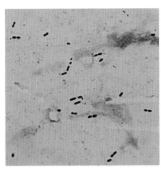

Plate 2 Pneumococci (*Streptococcus pneumoniae*) in a Gram-stained smear of sputum from a patient with pneumococcal pneumonia. The organisms are gram-positive and lancet shaped and appear mostly as diplococci.

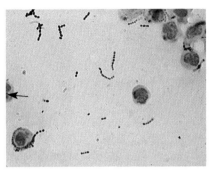

Plate 3 Streptococci (*Streptococcus pyogenes*) in a Gram-stained smear from an abscess. The organisms are gram-positive cocci in long chains. A few are intracellular in a polymorphonuclear leukocyte (arrow).

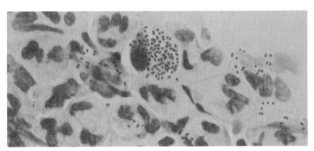

Plate 4 Gram-negative, bean-shaped diplococci (*Neisseria gonorrhoeae*) in a Gram-stained smear from a male urethral exudate. Many bacteria are seen in a single polymorphonuclear neutrophil. Other cells contain no or only a few diplococci.

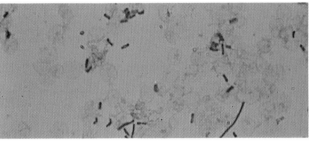

Plate 5 Gram-negative bacilli (*Klebsiella pneumoniae*) in a Gram-stained smear of a patient's blood culture. The organisms vary in length from short (coccobacillary) to long and filamentous. This variation is known as *pleomorphism*.

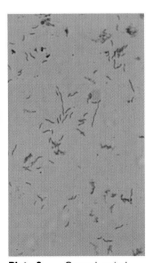

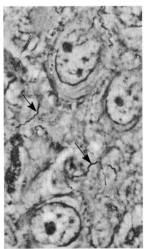

Plate 6 Curved, spiral, gram-negative bacilli (*Campylobacter jejuni*) in a Gram stain from a culture. Some bacteria line up to form spirillalike chains. Courtesy Dr. E. J. Bottone.

Plate 7 Spirochetes (*Treponema pallidum*) in a stained preparation from skin. A silver stain has been used, which makes the organisms appear black (arrows). Courtesy Dr. E. J. Bottone.

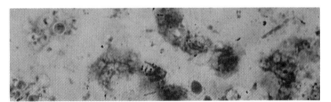

Plate 8 Acid-fast bacilli (*Mycobacterium tuberculosis*) in an acid-fast stain of sputum from a patient with tuberculosis. The acid-fast bacilli appear as red, beaded rods against a blue background. With this stain, inflammatory cells appear blue.

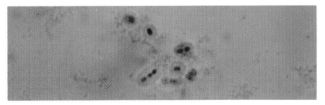

Plate 9 The quellung reaction in which pneumococcal cells have been treated with pneumococcal antiserum. The pneumococcal capsule (seen as a halo around the bacteria) appears to swell and is sharply demarcated. Compare with colorplate 28. Courtesy Dr. E. J. Bottone.

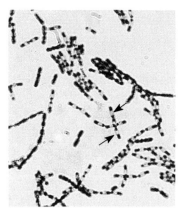

Plate 10 Gram-positive bacilli with endospores (*Bacillus* sp.). The endospores appear as clear areas within the gram-positive vegetative bacterial cell (arrows).

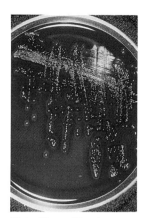

Plate 11 *Streptococcus pyogenes* growing on a blood agar plate. The clear areas of red cell lysis surrounding the punctate colonies (beta-hemolysis) are caused by the organism's streptolysin enzyme. Courtesy Dr. E. J. Bottone.

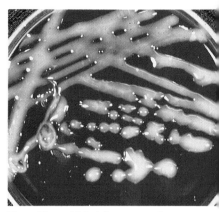

Plate 12 *Klebsiella pneumoniae* colonies growing on a blood agar plate. The organism produces a large capsule that gives a mucoid appearance to the colonies. Compare with colorplate 20. Courtesy Dr. E. J. Bottone.

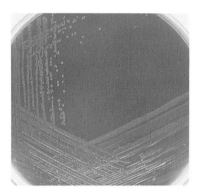 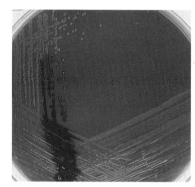

Plate 13 *Neisseria gonorrhoeae* colonies growing on a chocolate agar plate. The plate on the left shows gray, isolated colonies. On the right, a drop of oxidase reagent has been added to one area of the plate. The colonies in this area become deep purple, signifying a positive oxidase reaction.

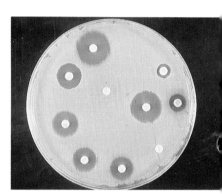

Plate 14 A disk diffusion antimicrobial susceptibility test. If the clear zones of growth inhibition around disks are of a certain diameter the organism is susceptible to the antimicrobial agent in the disk.

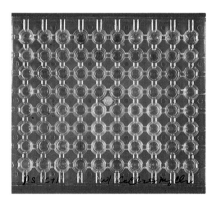

Plate 15 A microdilution susceptibility test. A series of concentrations of several different antimicrobial agents are contained in the tray wells. The organism tested in this tray (*Pseudomonas aeruginosa*) produces a soluble green pigment naturally. Therefore, the organism is growing in each well that appears green and is resistant to the particular antimicrobial agent concentration in that well.

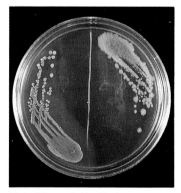

Plate 16 A MacConkey agar plate with *Escherichia coli* (pink, lactose-fermenting colonies) growing on the left-hand side and a *Salmonella* sp. (colorless, lactose nonfermenting colonies) on the right. Courtesy Dr. E. J. Bottone.

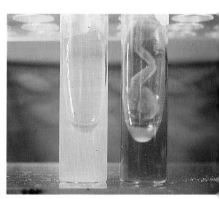

Plate 17 The urease test. The organism on the right produces the enzyme urease, which imparts a bright pink color (alkaline reaction) to the urea agar slant. The organism on the left does not produce urease. Courtesy Dr. E. J. Bottone.

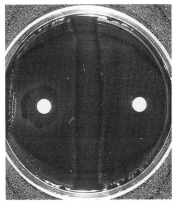

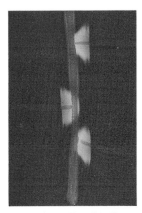

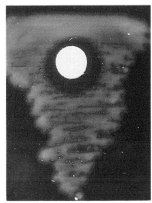

Plate 18   The bacitracin test. The zone of growth inhibition seen for the organism on the left (bacitracin susceptible) identifies it presumptively as a group A beta-hemolytic streptococcus (*Streptococcus pyogenes*). The organism on the right (bacitracin resistant) is a beta-hemolytic streptococcus other than *S. pyogenes*. Courtesy Dr. E. J. Bottone.

Plate 19   The CAMP test. When a group B streptococcus (*Streptococcus agalactiae*) is streaked at right angles to a hemolytic *Staphylococcus aureus* (long straight streak down middle of plate), areas of synergistic hemolysis in the shape of a beta-hemolytic arrow are formed. Courtesy Dr. E. J. Bottone.

Plate 20   The optochin test. A zone of inhibition forming around a disk containing optochin identifies this organism presumptively as *Streptococcus pneumoniae*. Notice the incomplete zone of hemolysis (alpha-hemolysis) around the organism growth and the colonies' mucoid appearance (compare with colorplate 12). Courtesy Dr. E. J. Bottone.

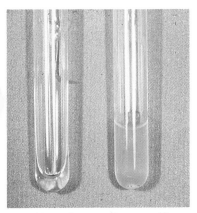

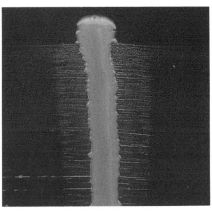

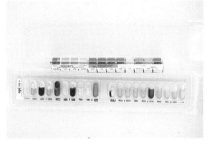

Plate 21   The coagulase test. The tube of plasma on the right was inoculated with *Staphylococcus aureus*. A solid clot has formed in this tube as compared with the still liquid plasma in the uninoculated tube on the left. Courtesy Dr. E. J. Bottone.

Plate 22   The satellite test. Colonies of *Haemophilus influenzae*, which requires both X factor (hemin) and V factor (a coenzyme, NAD), grow only around *Staphylococcus aureus* colonies on a blood agar plate. The blood provides the needed X factor, and the staphylococcus the V factor.

Plate 23   Rapid bacterial identification in the Enterotube II (top) and API strip (bottom). Many reactions are tested simultaneously, therefore, a definitive identification can be obtained after overnight incubation. The API strip has been inoculated with *Klebsiella pneumoniae*. The Enterotube II is uninoculated.

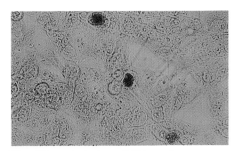

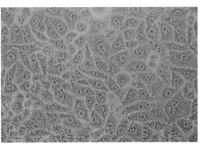

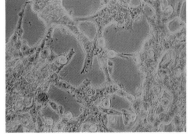

Plate 24   Inclusions of *Chlamydia trachomatis* in McCoy cell culture. The glycogen-containing inclusions stain dark brown when the cells are treated with an iodine solution. Courtesy Dr. E. J. Bottone.

Plate 25   Cell culture of adenovirus. The uninoculated cells on the left form an even monolayer (one cell thick) in the culture tube. Once the cells are infected with the virus (right), they undergo a characteristic cytopathic effect, becoming enlarged, granular in appearance, and aggregated into irregular clusters. This preparation has been photographed through a phase-contrast microscope. Courtesy Dr. E. J. Bottone.

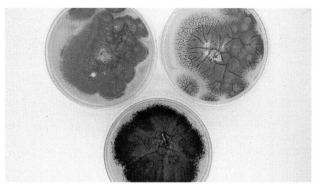

Plate 26 Colonies of three *Aspergillus* species. Some molds may be recognized by the color of the conidia (spores) they produce. Clockwise from left: *A. flavus* (yellow), *A. fumigatus* (smoky gray-green), *A. niger* (black).

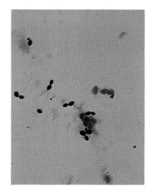

Plate 27 Gram stain of yeast cells (*Candida albicans*). Left, gram-positive budding cells from a sputum smear; right, yeast from a culture of patient's blood. Notice that long, filamentous, irregularly staining hyphae have formed.

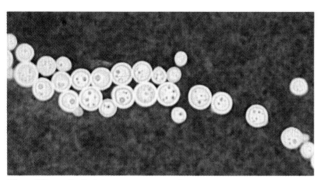

Plate 28 India ink preparation of *Cryptococcus neoformans*. These yeast cells from the cerebrospinal fluid of an AIDS patient are surrounded by a capsule that is demarcated by the suspension of charcoal particles in the India ink. Compare with colorplate 9. Courtesy Dr. E. J. Bottone.

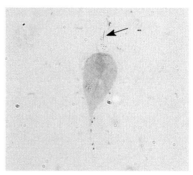

Plate 29 *Trichomonas vaginalis* in a gram stain of vaginal secretions. At least one flagellum (arrow) can be clearly seen. Most other parasites do not stain with the gram stain.

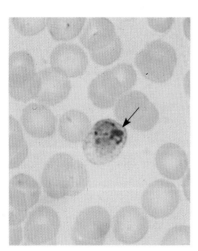

Plate 30 *Plasmodium vivax* trophozoite in a red blood cell (arrow). The red and blue malarial parasite causes the red blood cell to enlarge and to show characteristic stippling (Schüffner's dots). Courtesy Dr. E. J. Bottone.

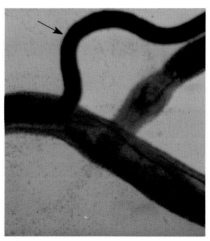

Plate 31 *Schistosoma mansoni*, a blood fluke. The smaller female adult (arrow) lives in the gynecophoral canal of the male where it attains sexual maturity. Courtesy Dr. E. J. Bottone.

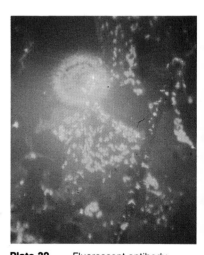

Plate 32 Fluorescent antibody preparation of *Legionella pneumophila*. A smear of patient's tracheal aspirate has been treated with *L. pneumophila* antibody conjugated with a fluorescent dye. The brightly fluorescing *Legionella* bacilli stand out against the dark background when viewed microscopically with an ultraviolet light source. Courtesy Dr. E. J. Bottone.

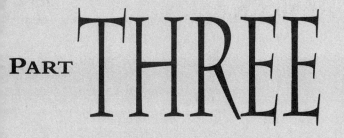

PART **THREE**   **Diagnostic Microbiology in Action**

General Considerations

The laboratory diagnosis of infectious disease **begins with the collection of a clinical specimen for examination and culture** (the *right one,* collected at the *right* time, transported in the *right* way to the *right* laboratory). It continues in the laboratory with the use of well-chosen techniques and methods for rapid isolation and identification of any pathogenic microorganisms the specimen may contain. In this part of the manual, we shall see how specimens from various parts of the body are cultured, what normal flora they may contain, and how the most usual pathogens are recognized. An understanding of the flow, sequence, and timing of the work is important to those involved in the care of patients with infectious diseases.

This understanding leads to an appreciation of how interim, preliminary information is valuable for patient management before the laboratory report is completed. Also, the terminology of laboratory reports must be understood, so that their significance can be recognized immediately. For example, you will learn why a report of an "alpha-hemolytic *Streptococcus*" in a throat culture has little, if any, importance, whereas a finding of "beta-hemolytic *Streptococcus,* group A" may have great significance. If a stool, urine, or blood culture report lists *Salmonella typhi* among the laboratory findings, you will know that the patient in question has a serious, readily transmissible disease, and that precautions designed to prevent the spread of the disease must be instituted.

These exercises do not present comprehensive details of clinical microbiology. Rather, they are designed to familiarize you with principles that you can apply in your professional work.

Microbiology at the Bedside

Collection and Transport of Clinical Specimens for Culture

Proper collection of an appropriate clinical specimen is the first step in obtaining an accurate laboratory diagnosis of an infectious disease. Applying your knowledge of microbiology at the bedside, where the specimen is collected, is as important as it is in the laboratory, for an inadequate specimen may lead to an inadequate diagnosis.

The following general rules apply to the collection and transport of any specimen for culture:

1. Strict aseptic technique must be used throughout the procedure.
2. Wash your hands before and after the collection.
3. Collect the specimen at the *optimum* time, as ordered by the physician. The timing of collection in relation to the patient's symptoms may determine whether the causative organism will be recovered in culture. (For example, spinal fluid from a case of suspected meningitis, blood from a patient with typhoid fever or pneumococcal pneumonia, or urine from an intermittent shedder of tubercle bacilli who has renal tuberculosis may be *negative* in culture if specimen collection is not timed well.)
4. Make certain the specimen is *representative* of the infectious process. If pneumonia is suspected, *sputum,* not saliva, must be collected. Pus from an abscess or wound should be collected from the depth, not the surface, of the lesion.
5. Collect or place the specimen aseptically in an appropriate, sterile container provided by the laboratory *for this purpose* and no other. If the specimen is contaminated in the process, it may be useless.
6. After collection, make certain the *outside* of the specimen container is clean and uncontaminated. If the container has been soiled on the outside, wipe it carefully with an effective disinfectant, so that it will not be a source of infection for those who will handle it further.
7. Make certain the container is tightly closed so that its contents cannot leak out during transport to the laboratory.
8. Check whether enough material has been collected for the laboratory to perform all tests requested.
9. Label and date the container. Attach a laboratory request slip that has been completely and legibly filled in with all necessary information, including the suspected clinical diagnosis.
10. Arrange for immediate transport of the specimen to the appropriate laboratory. Keep in mind that many pathogenic microorganisms are delicate and do not adjust well to environmental conditions outside the body. They may die if not *cultured* and incubated promptly. They may not survive if the specimen is either refrigerated or incubated *prior* to culture.
11. *Wash your hands.*

Precautions for Handling Specimens or Cultures

Remember that clinical specimens are ordered for culture because infectious disease is suspected. Whether it is an actual specimen or one simulated in the classroom laboratory, *any* specimen should be handled as though it contains living, pathogenic microorganisms and with the same respect as a culture.

In 1985, the Centers for Disease Control (CDC) developed a strategy now referred to as "*universal precautions*" to address concerns about transmission of human immunodeficiency virus (HIV, the agent of acquired immune deficiency syndrome or AIDS) in the health care setting. The concept of universal precautions stresses that "*all patients should be assumed to be infectious for HIV and other bloodborne pathogens.*" Thus, in the hospital or other health care setting, these precautions should be followed when workers are exposed to blood, certain other body fluids (amniotic, pericardial, peritoneal, pleural, synovial, cerebrospinal), semen and vaginal secretions, or any body fluid visibly contaminated with blood. Because HIV (and hepatitis) transmission has not been documented from exposure to other body fluids (feces, nasal secretions, sputum, sweat, tears, urine, and vomitus), universal precautions do not apply to these fluids nor to saliva, except in the dental setting where saliva is likely to be contaminated with blood. To minimize the risks of acquiring HIV while performing job duties, workers may need to use gloves, masks, and protective clothing, which provide a barrier between the worker and the exposure source. Precautions should always be taken to avoid needle-stick injuries, and hands should be washed thoroughly if contaminated with blood, other body fluids to which universal precautions apply, or potentially contaminated articles. Equipment, surfaces, and blood spills should be thoroughly and properly disinfected. In the clinical microbiology laboratory, gloves are always worn when handling patient specimens and blood cultures but not other materials already in culture. Gowns, masks, and protective eyewear are available for procedures in which there is a risk of HIV transmission.

In the following exercises, you will be seeing and handling cultures of microorganisms that might be found in clinical specimens. Read again the "Safety Procedures and Precautions" stated in Part 1, Section I, pages 3–4, as well as the "General Laboratory Directions" on pages 4–5. Note that any microorganism is potentially pathogenic if given some special opportunity to enter into the body. Learn to respect them all.

An understanding of the rules for laboratory procedures and conduct provides the basis for laboratory safety. Correctly followed, these rules are better guides than vague fears. In fact, the laboratory, where microorganisms are understood and controlled, may be safer than a hospital, home, or public place where infection exists but is unrecognized.

The following rules are restated for emphasis:

1. No eating, drinking, or smoking in the laboratory.
2. Wash your hands carefully before and after each session.
3. Use disinfectant to keep your bench top clean.
4. Keep your bench area free of clutter.
5. Never put contaminated items (loops, pipettes) down on the bench.
6. Tie long hair back out of the way.
7. Conduct yourself quietly.
8. Never take cultures out of the laboratory.
9. If a culture is spilled or broken, do not panic. Flood the area with disinfectant and call the instructor.
10. Be assured that microorganisms do not fly, swim, or bombard. They can be controlled by good technique.

Normal Flora of the Body

Under normal circumstances, the human skin and mucous membranes (exterior or interior) are sterile only during intrauterine development. From the moment of passage through the birth canal and into the outer world, superficial tissues come in contact with microorganisms, begin to be colonized by them, and remain so throughout life. Ordinarily, this state of affairs is harmless, unnoticeable, and even beneficial. The microorganisms that normally colonize skin and membranes are called "saprophytes" because they live on dead tissue and, except under unusual circumstances, do not invade living cells. They are also called "commensals" because they "eat together" with their host in a state of harmony. Indeed, commensalistic colonizers often perform useful functions for the human host, by clearing away dead cellular debris, by producing metabolic substances that are of use to host cells (referred to as mutualism), and by competing with intruding microorganisms of potential pathogenicity.

As human tissue structure and function change with age, activities, and environmental influences, the microbial "normal flora" changes also, as different species find life more or less untenable under new host conditions. *Everything* that influences the host also influences the host's normal flora, including stage of physiological development, food or medications, climate, clothing, and living habits.

Only the most superficial body tissues are colonized by saprophytic microorganisms. The defenses of the healthy body prevent invasion of commensal organisms into deep tissues. "Superficial" tissues include not only the skin, but mucous membranes that extend from the surface inward, lining the respiratory, intestinal, and genital tracts. Interior membrane surfaces are usually particularly rich with microbial growth because they offer warmth, moisture, and nutrient secretions. The flora of different areas of membranes and of skin varies according to conditions of growth offered.

Infectious diseases are usually established when pathogenic microorganisms enter by invading body surface tissues (respiratory, intestinal, genital or urogenital tracts, or skin). *Direct* entry of deep tissues is accomplished only by trauma of some kind, inflicted by a biting insect, contaminated needle or instruments, or other penetrating object.

In the exercises of Part 3 we shall study some of the normal flora of the body, as well as some of the pathogenic bacteria that cause infectious disease.

SECTION VII

Principles of Diagnostic Microbiology

Culture of Clinical Specimens;
Identifying Isolated Microorganisms

For more than 100 years, from the time Louis Pasteur (1822–1895) reformulated the germ theory of disease, and Robert Koch (1843–1910) developed his famous "postulates" for establishing the relationship of microbes to disease, clinical microbiologists have been at work isolating and identifying the causative agents of infections. In principle, most of the methods in common use today are the same as those developed a century ago. However, a great deal has been learned about the biochemistry of microbial metabolism, and this knowledge has greatly improved the speed, ease, and precision with which today's microbiologists identify pathogenic microorganisms.

The principles of diagnostic microbiology are based on an understanding of the metabolic behavior of microorganisms in culture. Prompt, accurate recognition of pathogenic species is achieved by choosing appropriate culture media for isolating these organisms from clinical specimens, and by selecting proper tests for determining their characteristic metabolic activities.

EXERCISE 16   Primary Media for Isolation of Microorganisms

Reference: Morello, Mizer, Wilson, and Granato, Microbiology in Patient Care, *5th edition, 1994.*
Chapter 4.

As we have seen, many clinical specimens contain a mixed flora of microorganisms. When these specimens are set up for culture, if only one isolation plate were inoculated, a great deal of time would be spent in subculturing and sorting through the bacterial species that grow out. Instead, the microbiologist uses several types of primary media (i.e., a battery) to culture the specimen initially. In general, the primary battery has three basic purposes, accomplished simultaneously: (1) to culture all bacterial species present and see which, if any, predominates; (2) to differentiate species by certain characteristic responses to ingredients of the culture medium; and (3) to selectively encourage growth of those species of interest while suppressing the normal flora.

The basic medium used to support the total flora of a clinical specimen contains agar enriched with blood and other nutrients required by pathogenic microorganisms. The blood is obtained from animal sources (sheep or rabbits, sometimes horses). Both the plasma and the red cells of blood provide excellent enrichment. The use of human blood (usually obtained from outdated collections in blood banks) in culture media is not recommended, because it may contain substances such as antimicrobial agents, antibodies, and anticoagulants that are either inhibitory to the growth of fastidious microorganisms or interfere with differential reactions.

In addition to basic nutrients, *differential media* contain one or more components, such as a particular carbohydrate, that can be used by some microorganisms but not by others. If the microorganism uses the component during the incubation period, a change occurs in an indicator that is also included in the medium (see colorplate 16).

Selective media contain one or more components that suppress the growth of some microorganisms without seriously affecting the ability of others to grow. Such media may also contain ingredients for differentiating among the species that do survive.

When a battery of culture media such as described above is streaked simultaneously upon receipt of a clinical specimen, the first results indicate what types of bacteria are present, in general how many, and which did or did not use the differential carbohydrate. Also, the species of particular interest on the selective medium (if that species was present in the specimen) has been singled out and differentiated. Thus, the process of identification of isolated pathogens is already well under way after 24 hours of incubation of specimen cultures.

Table 16.1 summarizes the most commonly used enriched, selective, and differential media, indicating their purpose as primary media for the isolation of microorganisms. The table should be reviewed before performing the exercise.

Table 16.1 Culture Media for the Isolation of Pathogenic Bacteria from Clinical Specimens

Media	Classification	Selective and Differential Agent(s)	Type of Organisms Isolated
Chocolate agar	Enriched	1% hemoglobin and supplements	Most fastidious pathogens such as *Neisseria* and *Haemophilus*
Blood agar plates (BAP)	Enriched and differential	5% defibrinated sheep blood	Almost all bacteria; differential for hemolytic organisms
Mannitol salt agar (MSA)	Selective and differential	7.5% NaCl and mannitol for isolation and identification of most *S. aureus* strains	Staphylococci and micrococci
MacConkey agar	Selective and differential	Lactose, bile salts, neutral red, and crystal violet	Gram-negative enteric bacilli
Eosin methylene blue agar (EMB)	Selective and differential	Lactose, eosin Y, and methylene blue	Gram-negative enteric bacilli
Hektoen enteric agar (HE)	Selective and differential	Lactose, sucrose, bile salts, ferric ammonium sulfate, sodium thiosulfate, bromthymol blue, acid fuchsin	*Salmonella* and *Shigella* species (enteric pathogens)
Phenylethyl alcohol agar (PEA)	Selective	Phenylethyl alcohol (inhibits gram negatives)	Gram-positive bacteria
Colistin nalidixic acid agar (CNA)	Selective	Colistin and nalidixic acid (inhibit gram negatives)	Gram-positive bacteria
Modified Thayer-Martin agar (MTM)	Selective	Hemoglobin, growth factors, and antimicrobial agents	Pathogenic *Neisseria* species

Purpose	To observe the response of a mixed bacterial flora in a clinical specimen to a battery of primary media
Materials	Nutrient agar plates Blood agar plates Eosin methylene blue agar plates (EMB) Mannitol salt agar plates (MSA) Simulated fecal suspension, containing *Escherichia coli, Pseudomonas aeruginosa,* and *Staphylococcus epidermidis* Demonstration plates: Mannitol salt plate streaked with *Staphylococcus aureus* on one side (pure culture), *Escherichia coli* on the other (pure culture) Eosin methylene blue plate streaked with *Staphylococcus aureus* and *Escherichia coli,* as above

Procedures

1. Inoculate the simulated fecal specimen on nutrient agar, blood agar, EMB, and MSA plates. Streak each plate for isolation of colonies. Incubate at 35°C.
2. Make a Gram stain of the fecal suspension and examine it.
3. Examine the demonstration plates (do not open them) and record your observations.

Results

1. Demonstration plates:
   a. Describe the appearance of *S. aureus* on
      Mannitol salt agar

      EMB agar

   b. Describe the appearance of *E. coli* on
      Mannitol salt agar

      EMB agar

2. Simulated fecal specimen cultures:

Medium	Gross Morphology of Each Colony Type	Gram-Stain Reaction of Each Colony Type	Microscopic Morphology of Each Colony Type

Questions

1. Define a *differential medium* and discuss its purpose.

2. Define a *selective medium* and describe its uses.

3. Why is MacConkey agar selective as well as differential?

4. Why is blood agar useful as a primary isolation medium?

5. How can one distinguish *E. coli* from *P. aeruginosa* on

   Nutrient agar? _____

   Blood agar? _____

   EMB agar? _____

6. What is the major difference between Modified Thayer-Martin (MTM) and chocolate agar? When would you use MTM rather than chocolate agar?

7. If you wanted to isolate *S. aureus* from a pus specimen containing a mixed flora, what medium would you choose to get results most rapidly? Why?

8. What is the value of making a Gram stain directly from a clinical specimen?

9. Why is aseptic technique important in the laboratory? In patient care?

EXERCISE 17 Some Metabolic Activities of Bacteria

Reference: Morello, Mizer, Wilson, and Granato, Microbiology in Patient Care, 5th edition, 1994. Chapters 3, 4.

Microbial metabolic processes are complex, but they permit the microbiologist to distinguish among microorganisms grown in culture. Bacteria, especially, are identified by inoculating pure, isolated colonies into media that contain one or more specific biochemicals. The biochemical reactions that take place in the culture can then be determined by relatively simple indicator reagents, included in the medium or added to the culture later.

Some bacteria ferment simple carbohydrates, producing acidic, alcoholic, or gaseous end products. Many different species are distinguished on the basis of the carbohydrates they do or do not attack, as well as by the nature of end products formed during fermentation. Still others break down more complex carbohydrates, such as starch. The nature of products formed in amino acid metabolism also provides information as to the identification of bacterial species. The production of visible pigments distinguishes certain types of bacteria.

Working with pure cultures freshly isolated from clinical specimens, the microbiologist uses a carefully selected battery of special media to identify their outstanding biochemical properties.

EXPERIMENT 17.1 Simple Carbohydrate Fermentations

Media for testing carbohydrate fermentation are often prepared as tubed broths, each tube containing a small inverted "fermentation" (or Durham) tube for trapping any gas formed when the broth is inoculated and incubated. Each broth contains essential nutrients, a specific carbohydrate, and a color reagent to indicate a change in pH if acid is produced in the culture (the broth is adjusted to a neutral pH when prepared). Organisms that grow in the broth but do not ferment the carbohydrate produce no change in the color of the medium, and no gas is formed. Some organisms may produce acid products in fermenting the sugar, but no gas, whereas others may form both acid and gas. In some cases, organisms that do not ferment the carbohydrate use the protein nutrients in the broth, thereby producing alkaline end products, a result that is also evidenced by a change in indicator color.

Purpose	To distinguish bacterial species on the basis of simple carbohydrate fermentation
Materials	Tubed phenol red glucose broth ⎫ Tubed phenol red lactose broth ⎬ with Durham tubes Tubed phenol red sucrose broth ⎭ Slant cultures of *Escherichia coli, Serratia marcescens, Pseudomonas aeruginosa,* and *Proteus vulgaris*

Procedures

1. Inoculate growth from each of the four cultures into separate tubes of each of the three carbohydrate broths. Be certain no bubbles are inside the Durham tubes before inoculation.
2. Label each of the 12 inoculated tubes with the name of the carbohydrate it contains and the name of the bacterial culture.
3. Incubate at 35°C for 24 hours.

Results

Record your results in the following table. Use the following symbols to indicate specific changes observed in the broths:

A = acid production
K = alkaline color change
N = neutral (no change in color)
G = gas formation

Name of Organism	Glucose	Lactose	Sucrose

EXPERIMENT 17.2   Starch Hydrolysis

Some microorganisms split apart (hydrolyze) large organic molecules and then use the component parts in further metabolic processes. Starch is a polysaccharide that is hydrolyzed by some bacteria. When iodine is added to the *intact* starch molecule, a blue-colored complex forms. If starch is hydrolyzed by bacterial enzymes, however, it is broken down to simple sugars (glucose and maltose) that do not complex with iodine, and no color reaction is seen.

   The medium for this test is a nutrient agar containing starch, prepared in a petri plate. The organism to be tested is streaked on the plate. When the culture has grown, the plate is flooded with Gram's iodine solution. The medium turns blue in all areas where the starch remains intact. The areas of medium surrounding organisms that have hydrolyzed the starch remain clear and colorless.

Purpose	To distinguish bacterial species on the basis of starch hydrolysis
Materials	Starch agar plates Slant cultures of *Escherichia coli, Pseudomonas aeruginosa,* and *Bacillus subtilis* Gram's iodine solution

Procedures

1. Take one starch plate, invert it, and with your marking pencil mark three triangular compartments on the back of the dish.
2. Inoculate one section of the agar with *E. coli,* using back-and-forth streaking; another section with *B. subtilis;* and the third with *P. aeruginosa.*
3. Label each section of the plate on the back of the dish with the name of the organism streaked in that area.
4. Incubate 24 to 48 hours at 35°C.
5. When the cultures have grown, drop Gram's iodine solution onto the plate until the entire surface is lightly covered.

Name _____ Class _____ Date _____

Results

Read and record your results in the following table.

Name of Organism	Color around Colony	Positive or Negative for Starch Hydrolysis

EXPERIMENT **17.3**　**Production of Indole and Hydrogen Sulfide, and Motility**

Indole is a by-product of the metabolic breakdown of the amino acid tryptophan used by some microorganisms. The presence of indole in a culture grown in a medium containing tryptophan can be readily demonstrated by adding Kovac's reagent to the culture. If indole is present, it combines with the reagent to produce a brilliant red color. If it is *not* present, there will be no color except that of the reagent itself. This test is of great value in the battery used to identify enteric bacteria, as you will see in Exercises 24 and 25.

Hydrogen sulfide is produced when amino acids containing sulfur are metabolized by microorganisms. If the medium contains metallic ions, such as lead, bismuth, or iron (in addition to an appropriate amino acid), the hydrogen sulfide formed during growth combines with the metallic ions to form a metal sulfide that blackens the medium.

The most convenient medium for testing for indole and/or hydrogen sulfide production is SIM medium (SIM is an acronym for *sulfide, indole,* and *motility*). This is a tubed semisolid agar that can also be used to demonstrate bacterial motility. It is inoculated by stabbing the wire loop (or preferably a straight wire inoculating needle) straight down the middle of the agar to about one-fourth the depth of the medium and withdrawing the wire along the same path.

Purpose	To observe how a single medium can be used to test for three distinguishing features of bacterial growth
Materials	Tubes of SIM medium Xylene Kovac's reagent 5-ml pipettes Bulb or other pipette aspiration device Slant cultures of *Escherichia coli, Proteus vulgaris,* and *Klebsiella pneumoniae* Broth cultures of *Escherichia coli, Proteus vulgaris,* and *Klebsiella pneumoniae*

Procedures

1. Inoculate growth from each of the three slant cultures into separate tubes of SIM medium. Stab the inoculating wire straight down through the agar for a distance of about one-fourth of its depth. Quickly withdraw the wire along the same path (do not move it around in the agar).
2. Incubate the tubes at 35°C for 24 hours.
3. Examine the tubes for evidence of hydrogen sulfide production (browning or blackening of the medium). Record results.

Figure 17.1 Semisolid agar tubes stabbed for motility test. (a) Pattern of growth of a motile organism. The entire medium is turbid with the growth of the organism, which has moved away from the stab line. (b) Pattern of growth of a nonmotile organism. Only the stab line is turbid with growth.

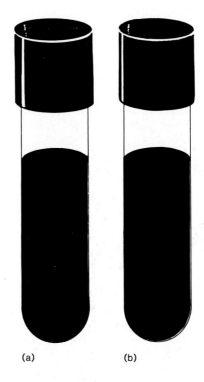

(a)   (b)

4. Examine the tubes for evidence of motility of the organism. A motile species grows away from the line of stab into the surrounding agar. Lines of growth, or even general turbidity, can be seen throughout the tube. The growth of a nonmotile organism is restricted to the path of the stab (fig. 17.1). Record your observations.
5. Set up a hanging-drop or wet-mount preparation of each broth culture to confirm results observed in SIM medium for motility (see Exercise 3 for procedure).
6. Perform the Kovac test for indole as follows:
   a. Using a pipette bulb or other aspiration device, pipette 1 ml of xylene into the SIM tube (it will layer over the top surface of the agar).
   b. Pipette 1 ml of Kovac's reagent in the same way as you did the xylene and add it to the SIM tube.
   c. Observe the color of the xylene layer, and record.

Results

Record your observations and results in the following table.

Name of Organism	Sulfide	Indole	Motility	
			SIM Medium	Hanging Drop

Questions

1. What is the color of phenol red at an acid pH?

2. What is the function of a Durham tube?

3. Why is iodine used to detect starch hydrolysis?

4. Name one indole-positive organism.

5. How is indole produced in SIM medium? How is it detected?

6. How is hydrogen sulfide demonstrated in this medium?

7. Name two methods for determining bacterial motility.

8. Why is it essential to have pure cultures for biochemical tests?

9. Could a pH-sensitive color indicator be used to reveal the presence of a contaminant in a fluid that should be sterile? Explain.

EXERCISE 18 Activities of Bacterial Enzymes

Reference: Morello, Mizer, Wilson, and Granato, Microbiology in Patient Care, 5th edition, 1994. Chapters 3, 4.

Enzymes are the most important chemical mediators of every living cell's activities. These organic substances catalyze, or promote, the uptake and use of raw materials needed for synthesis of cellular components or for energy. Enzymes are also involved in the breakdown of unneeded substances or of metabolic side products that must be eliminated from the cell and returned to the environment.

As catalysts, enzymes promote changes only in very specific substances or *substrates,* as they are often called. Thus, in the previous exercise, the changes produced in simple carbohydrates and in starch substrates were brought about by different, specific enzymes. We have seen the activity of an enzyme with a different kind of outcome, the breakdown of an antimicrobial agent (Exp. 15.3), but the principle is exactly the same. In the latter instance, the beta-lactam enzyme penicillinase brought about a change in the substrate penicillin.

Since enzymes appear to be limited to particular substrates, it follows that each bacterial cell must possess a large battery of different enzymes, each mediating a different metabolic process. They are identified in terms of the type of change produced in the substrate. In naming them, the suffix *-ase* is usually added to the name of the substrate affected. Thus, *urease* is an enzyme that degrades urea, *gelatinase* breaks down gelatin (a protein), *penicillinase* inactivates penicillin, and so on.

In this exercise, we shall see how many bacterial enzymes are demonstrated and how their recognition in bacterial cultures leads to identification of species.

EXPERIMENT 18.1 The Activity of Urease

Some bacteria split the urea molecule in two, releasing carbon dioxide and ammonia. This reaction, mediated by the enzyme urease, can be seen in culture medium prepared with urea added as the substrate. Phenol red is also added as a pH indicator. When bacterial cells that produce urease are grown in this medium, urea is degraded, ammonia is released, and the pH becomes alkaline. This pH shift is detected by a change in the indicator color from orange-pink to dark pink (see colorplate 17).

Rapid urease production is characteristic of *Proteus* species and of a few other enteric bacteria that at one time were classified in the *Proteus* genus. This simple test can be useful, therefore, in distinguishing these organisms from other bacteria that resemble them.

Purpose	To observe the activity of urease and to distinguish bacteria that produce it from those that do not
Materials	Tubes of urea broth Slant cultures of *Escherichia coli* and *Proteus vulgaris*

Procedures

1. Inoculate a tube of urea broth with *E. coli,* and another with the *Proteus* culture.
2. Incubate the tubes at 35°C for 24 hours.

Results

Record your observations:

Name of Organism	Color of Broth After Culture	Color of Broth Before Culture	Urease	
			Positive	Negative

EXPERIMENT **18.2**   **The Activity of Catalase**

Many bacteria produce the enzyme catalase, which breaks down hydrogen peroxide, liberating oxygen. The simple test for catalase can be very useful in distinguishing between organism groups.

Purpose	To observe bacterial catalase activity
Materials	3% hydrogen peroxide 5-ml pipettes Pipette bulb or other aspiration device Slant cultures of *Staphylococcus epidermidis* and *Enterococcus faecalis*

Procedures

1. Hold the slant culture of the *Staphylococcus* in an inclined position and pipette 0.5 ml of hydrogen peroxide onto the surface with the bacterial growth. Observe closely for the appearance of gas bubbles.
2. Repeat the procedure with the *Enterococcus* culture. Note whether oxygen is liberated and bubbling occurs.

Results

Describe your observations and state your conclusions:

Staphylococcus epidermidis:

Bubbling ————————— No bubbling ——————— Catalase positive ————— negative —————————————————

Enterococcus faecalis:

Bubbling ————————— No bubbling ——————— Catalase positive ————— negative —————————————————

EXPERIMENT **18.3**   **The Activity of Gelatinase**

Gelatin is a simple protein. When in solution, it liquefies at warm temperatures above 25°C. At room temperature or below it becomes solid. When bacteria that produce the enzyme gelatinase are grown in a gelatin medium, the enzyme breaks up the gelatin molecule and the medium cannot solidify even at cold temperatures. An alternative method for detecting gelatinase production is the use of X-ray film that is coated with a green gelatin emulsion. Organisms that produce gelatinase remove the emulsion from the strip.

Purpose	To observe the usefulness of a gelatinase test in distinguishing between bacterial species
Materials	Tubes of nutrient gelatin medium 1 × ¼-inch strips of exposed, undeveloped X-ray film Tubes containing 0.5 ml sterile saline Slant cultures of *Serratia marcescens* and *Providencia stuartii*

Procedures

1. Inoculate each of the two cultures into a separate tube of gelatin, stabbing the inoculating wire straight down through the solid column of medium.
2. Incubate the inoculated tubes and one *un*inoculated tube of gelatin medium at 35°C.
3. Inoculate each of the two cultures into a separate tube of 0.5 ml saline. The suspension should be very turbid.
4. Insert a strip of the X-ray film into each saline suspension.
5. Incubate the tubes at 35°C. Observe at 1, 2, 3, 4, and 24 hours for removal of the green gelatin emulsion from the strip with subsequent appearance of the transparent blue strip support.
6. After 24 hours, examine the nutrient gelatin tubes. The uninoculated control as well as the two inoculated cultures should be liquid. Place all three tubes in the refrigerator for 30 minutes. If at the end of this period all tubes are solidified, replace them in the incubator. If any tube is liquefied but the others are solid, record this result.
7. If tubes are reincubated, examine them every 24 hours, placing them in the refrigerator for 30 minutes each time, as in previous procedures.

Results

	Tube method	X-ray film method
Serratia marcescens:	Gelatinase positive ____ in ____ hours	Gelatinase positive ____ in ____ hours
	Gelatinase negative ____	Gelatinase negative ____
Providencia stuartii:	Gelatinase positive ____ in ____ hours	Gelatinase positive ____ in ____ hours
	Gelatinase negative ____	Gelatinase negative ____

EXPERIMENT 18.4   The Activity of Deoxyribonuclease (DNase)

Some microorganisms secrete an enzyme that attacks the deoxyribonucleic acid (DNA) molecule. This can be demonstrated by streaking a plated agar medium containing the substrate DNA with a culture of the organism that produces the enzyme. The uninoculated medium is opaque and remains so after the culture has grown. If the plate is then flooded with weak hydrochloric acid, a zone of clearing appears around colonies that have produced DNase. This clearing occurs because the large DNA molecule has been degraded by the enzyme, and the end products dissolve in the added acid. Intact DNA does not dissolve in weak acid but rather is precipitated by it; therefore, the medium in the rest of the plate, or around colonies that do *not* produce DNase, becomes more opaque.

Purpose	To distinguish bacterial species that do and do not produce DNase
Materials	One DNA agar plate
	Dropping bottle containing 1 *N* HCl
	Slant cultures of *Escherichia coli* and *Serratia marcescens*

Procedures

1. Make a mark on the bottom of the DNA plate dividing it in half.
2. Inoculate one side of the plate with *Escherichia coli* by making a single streak about 5 cm in length. Use a heavy inoculum.
3. Inoculate the other side of the plate with *Serratia marcescens,* in the same manner.
4. Incubate the plate at 35°C for 24 hours.
5. Examine the plate for growth.
6. Drop 1 *N* HCl onto the agar surface until it is thinly covered with acid.
7. Examine the areas around the growth on both sides of the plate for evidence of clearing or opacity.

Results

Make a diagram of your observations:

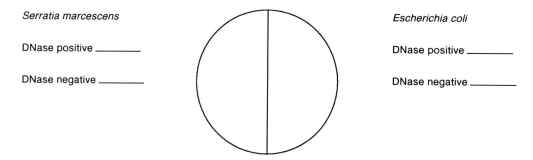

Serratia marcescens

DNase positive _____

DNase negative _____

Escherichia coli

DNase positive _____

DNase negative _____

EXPERIMENT 18.5   The Activity of a Deaminase

Most bacteria possess a battery of enzymes that specifically break down individual amino acids. In the process, the amine group on the molecule is removed and the amino acid is degraded, the reaction being known as *deamination*. The deaminases that effect this type of change are named for the particular amino acid substrate for which they are specific. In this experiment, we will see the effects of a phenylalanine deaminase (PDase) produced by some bacteria.

When the amino acid phenylalanine is incorporated into a culture medium in which PDase-producing bacteria are growing, the substrate is degraded to phenylpyruvic acid. The reaction is made visible by adding ferric ions, which react with the newly produced acid to form a green compound. The appearance of a green color in a medium that was colorless when inoculated is evidence of the activity of the deaminase.

Purpose	To observe the activity of PDase and to distinguish bacteria that produce it from those that do not
Materials	Slants of phenylalanine agar Dropping bottle containing 10% ferric chloride Slant cultures of *Escherichia coli* and *Providencia stuartii*

Procedures

1. Inoculate each of the two cultures on a separate slant of phenylalanine agar.
2. Incubate the new cultures at 35°C for 24 hours.
3. Examine the tubes for heavy growth. If it is adequate, run a few drops of 10% ferric chloride solution down the surface of each slant.
4. Observe the tubes for development of a green color.

Results

E. coli: Color _____ PDase positive _____ negative _____

Providencia stuartii: Color _____ PDase positive _____ negative _____

Questions

1. What is a catalyst?

2. Define an *enzyme* and a *substrate.* What is the value of enzyme tests in diagnostic microbiology?

3. What happens to urea in the presence of urease?

4. What is the substrate of the catalase reaction? Why are bubbles produced in a positive catalase test?

5. Why is gelatin liquefied in the presence of gelatinase?

6. Describe a positive DNase test.

7. What is a deaminase?

8. For each of the following enzymes, indicate one bacterial species that produces it:

Urease _____

Catalase _____

Gelatinase _____

Deoxyribonuclease _____

Phenylalanine deaminase _____

SECTION VIII

Microbiology of the Respiratory Tract

EXERCISE 19 Streptococci, Pneumococci, and Enterococci

*Reference: Morello, Mizer, Wilson, and Granato, Microbiology in Patient Care, 5th edition, 1994.
Chapters 6, 12, 19.*

The mucous membranes of the upper respiratory tract that are exposed to air and food (nose, throat, mouth) normally display a variety of aerobic and anaerobic bacterial species: gram-positive cocci (*Streptococcus, Staphylococcus,* and *Peptostreptococcus* species); gram-negative cocci (*Neisseria, Branhamella,* and *Veillonella* species); gram-positive bacilli (*Corynebacterium, Propionibacterium,* and *Lactobacillus* species); gram-negative bacilli (*Haemophilus* and *Bacteroides* species); and, sometimes, yeasts (*Candida* species).

This flora varies somewhat in various areas of the upper respiratory tract, the nasal membranes showing a predominance of staphylococci; the throat (pharyngeal membranes), the richest variety of species; sinus membranes, few if any organisms. The deeper reaches of the respiratory tract (trachea, bronchi, alveoli) are not readily colonized by microorganisms, because the ciliated epithelium of the upper membranes, together with mucous secretions, trap and move them upward and outward.

Usually the normal flora of the upper respiratory tract prevents entry and overgrowth of the membranes by transient microorganisms, some of which might be pathogenic and capable of invading respiratory lining cells or deeper tissues. If the *status quo* maintained by commensal organisms is disturbed (by changes in the condition of the host, by administration of antimicrobial agents to which the commensals are susceptible, or by unusual exposure to virulent, transient pathogens in large numbers), other microorganisms may then be able to colonize and invade the membranes.

EXPERIMENT 19.1 Isolation and Identification of Streptococci

The genus *Streptococcus* contains gram-positive cocci that characteristically are arranged in chains (see colorplate 3). There are a number of species of streptococci, some of which are normally found in the environment or among the normal flora of human skin and mucous membranes, particularly those of the upper respiratory tract. Certain species are more commonly associated with human infectious diseases than others.

Many streptococci have fastidious growth requirements; that is, they require blood-enriched media and a well-controlled atmosphere of incubation. Most are *facultatively aerobic* (grow well in air but also grow in the absence of oxygen), some *microaerophilic* (prefer reduced oxygen tension and also some increased CO_2), and some are *anaerobic* (grow only in the absence of oxygen). The latter are now placed in the genus *Peptostreptococcus* (see Exercise 28). An incubation temperature of 35°C is optimal for most streptococci.

A number of streptococcal species produce substances that destroy red blood cells; that is, they cause *lysis* of the cell wall with subsequent release of hemoglobin. Such substances are called *lysins,* or, more specifically, *hemolysins.* Many bacteria that are associated with human infection may be hemolytic. Certain strains of staphylococci, *Escherichia coli, Haemophilus,* some anaerobes, and many others also produce hemolytic substances, which are sometimes named for the organisms (e.g., *staphylolysin* or *streptolysin*). The activity of streptolysins or other hemolysins can be readily observed when the organisms are growing on a blood agar plate (see colorplate 11).

Different streptococci produce visibly different effects on the red cells in blood agar. Those that produce *incomplete* hemolysis and only partial clearing of the cells around colonies are called *alpha-hemolytic streptococci.* Many species of streptococci show alpha-hemolysis, and among them is a group that characteristically produces a distinct greening of the agar in the hemolytic zone. This group of alpha-hemolytic streptococci has traditionally been referred to as the *viridans* group (from the Latin word for *green*).

Species whose hemolysins cause *complete* destruction of red cells in the agar zones surrounding their colonies are said to be *beta-hemolytic.* When growing on blood agar, beta-hemolytic streptococci can be seen as small opaque or semitranslucent colonies surrounded by clear, glassy zones in an otherwise red opaque medium. One streptococcal hemolysin involved in this reaction is inhibited by oxygen. Its effect is seen best around subsurface colonies or when culture plates are incubated anaerobically. Some strains of staphylococci, *E. coli,* and other bacteria also may show beta-hemolysis as previously pointed out.

Strains of streptococci that do not produce hemolysins and are therefore *nonhemolytic* on blood agar are sometimes called *gamma* streptococci, but the term *nonhemolytic* is preferable.

Alpha-hemolytic and nonhemolytic streptococci abound among the normal flora of the human body, but they are sometimes also associated with infectious disease. In persons with damaged or abnormal heart valves, if these streptococci enter the bloodstream, they can travel to and colonize the damaged valve. The *infective endocarditis* that results is chronic and subacute (that is, moderate but progressive until treated) and sometimes referred to as *subacute bacterial endocarditis,* or *SBE.* Alpha-hemolytic and nonhemolytic streptococci may also be involved in urogenital or wound infections.

Beta-hemolytic streptococci are not commonly found among the normal flora of healthy individuals, although persons who are immune to their activities may be colonized by them. Certain strains of beta-hemolytic streptococci are more usually pathogenic—for animals as well as humans. When they damage human tissues, the body responds by pouring white blood cells into the area, as an accumulation of visible "pus." Because they cause this reaction, these streptococci are said to be *pyogenic,* or pus producing, and such virulent strains bear the species name *Streptococcus pyogenes.* Most notably, *S. pyogenes* is the cause of acute sore throat, scarlet fever, and erysipelas (a spreading skin infection). The infecting organisms produce a number of toxic substances (in addition to streptolysins) that may be disseminated through the body from the site of local infection in the upper respiratory tract. These toxins, or immunologic reactions against them or other streptococcal antigens, can affect the kidney (causing glomerulonephritis), the heart (causing acute rheumatic disease), the epithelium of the skin (as in scarlet fever rash), or deep skin tissues (erythema nodosum).

The numerous strains of pathogenic beta-hemolytic streptococci look alike in culture and cannot be distinguished readily by cultural methods. By immunological methods, they can be separated into several groups. Differences in their cell wall carbohydrate antigens (substances that stimulate humans or animals to produce antibodies) can be shown by immunological techniques, which place them in groups lettered from A through V. Immunological grouping has established the fact that most beta-hemolytic streptococci pathogenic for humans belong to *group A.* Because immunological grouping used to be time consuming, microbiologists sought and found a quicker method for presumptive identification of group A streptococci. In exploring their responses to antimicrobial agents, it was found that most group A beta-hemolytic streptococci are highly susceptible to low concentrations of the drug *bacitracin,* whereas those of other serological groups are more resistant to this agent.

Using bacitracin incorporated in a small filter paper disk placed on primary isolation or subculture plates, the microbiologist can presumptively identify group A streptococci. Strains that are susceptible to the drug are inhibited and do not grow in its presence. Strains of beta-hemolytic streptococci other than group A grow readily around the bacitracin disk (see colorplate 18). The filter paper is sometimes called an "A-disk." Streptococci that do not grow in its presence are reported as "beta-hemolytic streptococci, presumptive group A (by bacitracin)," meaning that they are not proven members of the pathogenic group serologically classed as A.

Commercial kits for serologically grouping streptococci are now available, which allow more precise identification of these microorganisms. The serological tests can be completed in from 10 to 30 minutes because they do not require an overnight incubation period, as does the bacitracin disk test. Thus, results are usually available the day after the patient's throat culture is obtained.

The basis of the two most common types of serological test kits for grouping streptococci is that antibody prepared against a streptococcal carbohydrate group antigen can be attached to the surface of either inert latex particles (*latex agglutination test*) or to cells of a special staphylococcus strain (*coagglutination test*). To perform the test, colonies of the suspicious organism growing on a blood agar plate (usually beta-hemolytic colonies that show gram-positive cocci in chains on Gram stain) are mixed with a solution that extracts the group antigen from the organism's cell wall. Following a short incubation period, a drop of the extraction solution is mixed with a drop of the antibody-coated latex or staphylococcal particles. Most often, the grouping kit contains individual antibody reagents for those streptococci that may be involved in human disease; that is, groups A, B, C, D, F, and G. Each antibody reagent is tested individually with the antigen extraction solution; the drops are mixed well on a special slide, and the mixtures are observed for clumping of the latex particles or staphylococci. Clumping (agglutination) signifies a positive reaction, a specific reaction that has occurred between the extracted group antigen and its related antibody, which is attached to the particle (fig. 19.1).

Figure 19.1 Diagram of a latex or coagglutination reaction. (a) When latex particles or staphylococcus cells that are coated with an antibody (for example, group A *Streptococcus* antibody) react with a specific antigen (group A *Streptococcus* antigen), the particles join together to form clumps that agglutinate on the test slide (lower left corner of (a)). In the control test that is always run in parallel on the same slide, the same antigen is mixed with latex or staphylococcal particles that are not coated with antibody, therefore, the particles remain in suspension and do not agglutinate. In diagram section (b), the antibody-coated particles do not react with the nonspecific antigen (for example, group B *Streptococcus* antigen), therefore, no clumps are formed, and the test as well as the control suspension shows no agglutination (lower left corner of (b)).

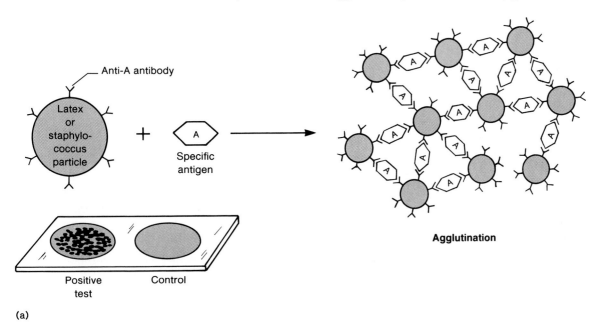

(a)

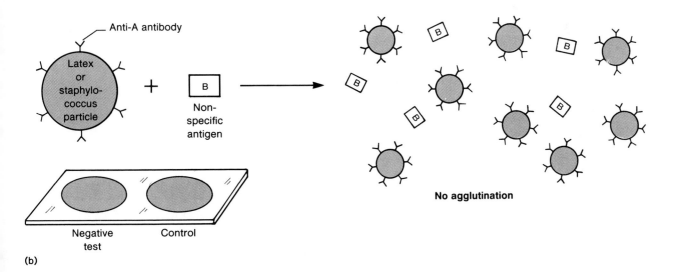

(b)

Latex and coagglutination reagents are commercially available for detecting microbial antigens that can be either extracted into solution (for example, streptococci), or are readily soluble (e.g., capsules of pneumococci, *Haemophilus influenzae,* and some *Neisseria meningitidis* groups). The last three organisms are those that most commonly cause bacterial meningitis, a serious and sometimes rapidly fatal disease. During an episode of meningitis, the capsular antigens of these bacteria are in solution in the patient's cerebrospinal fluid (CSF). These soluble antigens can be detected by mixing a drop of the CSF with latex or coagglutination reagents coated with antibodies (prepared by immunizing animals with the individual capsular antigens) and observing for clumping. In this way, a rapid diagnosis can be made before the organisms have grown out in culture. Antigen may also be detected in the patient's serum and urine.

In a few instances, microorganisms that belong to different genera have the same antigenic chemical structure on their surfaces; for example, a particular strain of *E. coli* (a gram-negative bacillus) shares the group B antigen of *N. meningitidis* (a gram-negative coccus). Because these surface antigens react with specific antibody reagents, it is possible to obtain a positive reaction when testing a microbial antigen other than the one to which the antibody reagent was prepared. In the previous example, a positive reaction would be seen when the *E. coli* is tested with *N. meningitidis* group B antibody. Therefore, when tests are performed directly on patient specimens rather than from colonies growing on a culture plate (where the colony morphology and Gram-stain reaction can be seen as well), the results must be interpreted with great caution because it is possible for these "false-positive" reactions to occur. Careful interpretation is especially important when no organisms are seen on direct Gram stain of the specimen.

Another type of rapid test is now available for identifying group A streptococci *directly* from a throat swab, without growing the organism in culture. Again the test relies on extracting streptococcal cell wall antigen, but from streptococci present on the throat swab rather than from organisms growing in culture. An antigen-antibody test that is more complex than simple latex agglutination or coagglutination is often used. This test is referred to as an *enzyme immunoassay* (EIA) or, sometimes, *enzyme-linked immunosorbent assay* (ELISA), because the antibody is attached to an enzyme. After a series of steps in which the extracted antigen and antibody-enzyme complex are allowed to react, the colorless substrate for the enzyme is added to "develop" the test. In a positive test, the enzyme hydrolyzes the substrate to form a colored end product that can be seen visually or detected by an instrument (fig. 19.2). This type of test is usually performed in clinics and in physicians' offices because it is rapid (10 to 30 minutes) and does not require culture expertise. However, for a positive test, a large number of organisms is needed on the swab. When negative results are obtained for patients with clinical evidence of pharyngitis, a throat swab for "strep" culture should always be sent to the clinical microbiology laboratory.

Among streptococcal diseases, those involving group A strains are most common and often severe. Laboratory diagnosis of most streptococcal disease thus depends on isolation and identification of beta-hemolytic streptococci proven serologically to belong to group A, or *presumptively* recognized as A-disk susceptible.

Strains of group B beta-hemolytic streptococci, once thought to cause animal disease primarily, are now known as agents of human disease as well. Group B strains colonize the female genital mucosa and are a potential infectious hazard for infants born of colonized mothers. Generalized infection or meningitis of the newborn caused by group B streptococci is serious and often fatal. Infected mothers also may develop grave postpartum group B disease. The final laboratory distinction of group A and B strains of beta-hemolytic streptococci is based on the serological method, but other tests may also distinguish between them. Group B strains are usually resistant to bacitracin, and, therefore, their growth is not inhibited by the A-disk and they produce a substance called the CAMP factor (see Exp. 19.2 and colorplate 19) that enhances the effect of beta-hemolysins possessed by some strains of *Staphylococcus aureus.*

Other streptococcal groups occasionally cause bloodstream infection or mild pharyngitis. The best method to differentiate them from groups A and B streptococci is by one of the serological agglutination tests just described.

In Experiment 19.1, we shall study some simple methods for isolating streptococci from clinical specimens and for presumptive and confirmatory identification of beta-hemolytic strains as group A. In Experiment 19.2, procedures for differentiating group B strains by the CAMP and serological tests will be followed.

Figure 19.2 Diagram of an enzyme immunoassay (EIA or ELISA). (a) A throat swab from a patient with streptococcal pharyngitis is placed in a tube with extraction solution, which extracts the group A antigen. (b) The extraction solution is then passed through a filter where the group A antigen attaches to its surface. (c) After a wash step, an antibody against the group A *Streptococcus,* which is linked to an enzyme, is added to the filter where it attaches to the group A antigen. (d) After another wash, a colorless substrate specific for the enzyme is added and is split to a colored end product when it comes in contact with the antibody-bound enzyme. (e) If an antigen other than group A was present, no antibody would bind. Unbound antibody would be washed away, and no color reaction would be seen.

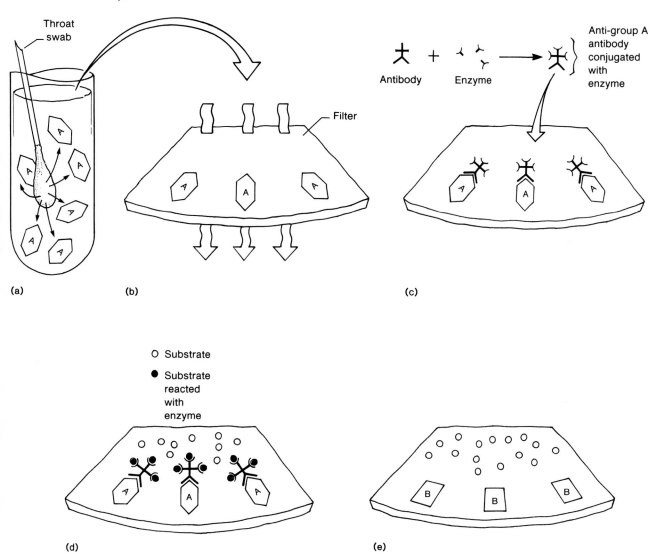

Purpose	To isolate and identify streptococci in culture
Materials	Sheep blood agar plate
	Simulated throat culture from a two-year-old child with acute tonsillitis
	Demonstration blood agar plate showing alpha-hemolytic, beta-hemolytic, and nonhemolytic strains of streptococci
	Demonstration plate showing response of two strains of beta-hemolytic streptococci to bacitracin A-disks
	Solution with extracted antigen of beta-hemolytic *Streptococcus* (prepared by instructor)
	Latex or coagglutination test kit for serological typing

Procedures

1. Inoculate and streak a blood agar plate with the simulated clinical specimen. Make a few stabs in the agar at the area of heaviest inoculum. Try not to stab to the bottom of the agar medium layer.
2. Incubate the plate at 35°C for 24 hours.
3. Examine the demonstration plates (but *do not open* them without supervision).
4. Following the manufacturer's directions, use the typing kit to identify serologically the beta-hemolytic isolate. Mix the antigen extract with a drop of each of the group A and group B latex or coagglutination reagents.
5. Observe both suspensions for evidence of agglutination.
6. Record your observations under Results (no. 7).·

Results

1. Describe the "patient's" throat culture results in the following table, after making Gram stains.

Morphology of Individual Colonies	Type of Hemolysis Displayed	Gram Reaction	Microscopic Morphology

2. Describe any differences in intensity of hemolysis around colonies growing on the agar surface and those pushed below the surface where you stabbed into the agar.

3. How would you report the culture in questions 1 and 2 to the physician?

4. Demonstration plate showing different types of hemolysis: describe your observations of

Alpha-hemolytic streptococci _____

_____

Beta-hemolytic streptococci _____

_____

Nonhemolytic streptococci _____

_____

5. Demonstration plate with A-disks: diagram your observations, indicating the position of the disks, areas of growth, and type of hemolysis.

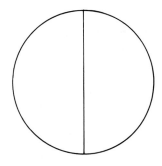

6. State your interpretation of the bacitracin disk results.

7. With which latex or coagglutination reagent did you obtain a positive result? Group _____

EXPERIMENT 19.2   The CAMP Test for Group B Streptococci

Group B streptococci can be distinguished from other beta-hemolytic streptococci by their production of a substance called the CAMP factor. This term is an acronym for the names of the investigators who first described the factor: *Christie, Atkins,* and *Munch-Petersen.* The substance is a peptide that acts together with the beta-hemolysin produced by some strains of *Staphylococcus aureus,* enhancing the effect of the latter on a sheep blood agar plate. This effect is sometimes referred to as *synergistic* hemolysis (see colorplate 19).

Purpose	To differentiate group B from group A streptococci by the effect of the group B CAMP factor and by a serological method
Materials	Demonstration sheep blood agar plate, streaked at separate points with *Staphylococcus aureus,* group B streptococci, and group A streptococci Solution with extracted antigen of beta-hemolytic *Streptococcus* (prepared by instructor) Latex or coagglutination test kit for serological typing

Procedures (Steps 1–4 to be followed by instructor)

1. With an inoculating loop, streak a strain of *S. aureus* down the center of a blood agar plate. (ATCC 25923 or other strain known to produce beta-hemolysin is used; 5% sheep blood agar is needed.)
2. On one side of the plate, inoculate a strain of group B *Streptococcus* by making a streak at a 90° angle, starting 5 mm away from the *S. aureus* and extending outward to the edge of the agar (see diagram).
3. On the other side of the plate, inoculate a strain of group A *Streptococcus*, again at a 90° angle from the *S. aureus*, as in step 2. This streak should not be directly opposite the group B inoculum (see diagram).
4. Incubate the plate aerobically at 35°C for 18 to 24 hours.
5. The student should confirm the isolate's identity by the serological test. Using the extracted antigen solution, follow the procedures in steps 4 and 5 of Experiment 19.1.

Results

1. Observe the area of hemolysis surrounding the *S. aureus* streak. At the point adjacent to the streak of group B streptococci, you should see an arrowhead-shaped area of increased hemolysis indicating production of the CAMP factor. There should be no change in the hemolytic zone adjacent to the streak of group A streptococci, most strains of which do not produce the CAMP factor.

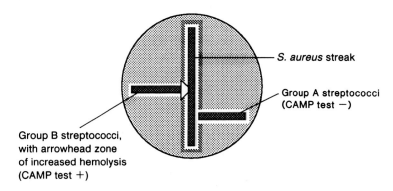

S. aureus streak

Group A streptococci
(CAMP test −)

Group B streptococci,
with arrowhead zone
of increased hemolysis
(CAMP test +)

2. Although most group A streptococci give a negative CAMP test, some have been reported to be positive, especially when the test plate has been incubated anaerobically rather than aerobically. The bacitracin disk test may be useful in distinguishing the latter from group B streptococci. Conversely, however, occasional strains of group B streptococci may be bacitracin susceptible. In such cases, a serological grouping method may be required for final identification. The following scheme may be followed by diagnostic laboratories reporting the results of these tests:

CAMP factor   + ⎱
Bacitracin   − ⎰ Presumptive group B streptococci

CAMP factor   − ⎱
Bacitracin   + ⎰ Presumptive group A streptococci

CAMP factor   + ⎱
Bacitracin   + ⎰ May be either group A or B; differentiate serologically

CAMP factor   − ⎱
Bacitracin   − ⎰ Not group A or group B streptococci (presumptive)

3. With which latex or coagglutination reagent did you obtain a positive result? Group _____

EXPERIMENT **19.3**   **Identification of Pneumococci**

Pneumococci are among the most important agents of bacterial pneumonia. Other microorganisms such as *Klebsiella pneumoniae* and *Haemophilus influenzae* (Exercise 21) or staphylococci (Exercise 20) may also be associated with serious pulmonary disease. Bacterial agents of pneumonia cause an acute inflammation of the bronchial and/or alveolar membranes. When the alveoli are severely involved, their thin membranes may be disrupted by hemorrhage of alveolar capillaries, and this, along with the multiplying infecting microorganisms, may cause them to collapse and consolidate. Consolidating pneumonia is always a serious clinical problem. Laboratory diagnosis is made primarily by identifying the causative agent in *sputum* sent for culture. Cultures of *blood* or *pleural fluid* may also be useful in diagnosis. In some patients, the organisms spread through the bloodstream to the central nervous system to cause meningitis. Pneumococci can then be isolated from the patient's CSF as well.

Pneumococci are classified in the genus *Streptococcus* as the species *pneumoniae*. They are gram-positive, lancet-shaped cocci that characteristically appear in pairs (diplococci) or in short chains (see colorplate 2). Like other streptococci, they are fastidious microorganisms and require blood-enriched media and microaerophilic conditions for primary isolation. They are alpha-hemolytic and usually produce greening of blood agar around their colonies. *Streptococcus pneumoniae* can be distinguished from other alpha-hemolytic streptococci because it is sensitive to bile salts and other surface active substances, including one known as optochin, and is lysed by them (see colorplate 20).

Another distinctive feature of pneumococci is their possession of a capsule, composed of a viscous polysaccharide. This slimy capsule serves to protect them from destruction by phagocytes that gather at sites of infection throughout the body to take them up. In the laboratory, the pneumococcal capsules are not readily demonstrated by usual staining techniques, but they can be made visible under the microscope by a serological technique known as the "quellung" reaction. *Quellung* is the German word for "swelling" and describes the microscopic appearance of pneumococcal or other bacterial capsules after their polysaccharide antigen has combined with a specific antibody present in a test serum from an immunized animal. As a result of this combination, and precipitation of the large, complex molecule formed, the capsule appears to swell, because of increased surface tension, and its outlines become clearly demarcated (see colorplate 9).

The capsular antigen can also be detected with latex and coagglutination antibody reagents. Colonies of suspected pneumococci growing on blood agar plates may be tested, or, depending on the disease severity, the soluble capsular antigen may be present in the patient's CSF, blood, and urine (the antigen, but not necessarily the organisms, is excreted from the body by the kidneys). Regardless of the results of direct antigen detection tests, sputum, blood, and CSF cultures should always be performed. In some instances, the antigen concentration in body fluids is too low to be detected, but cultures are positive.

Pneumococci are frequently found among the normal flora of the upper respiratory tract of healthy individuals. Their recovery in sputum cultures is not, of itself, conclusive evidence of pneumococcal disease. This finding must be correlated with the total picture of the patient's clinical illness.

Purpose	To identify pneumococci in culture
Materials	Dropping bottle containing 10% sodium desoxycholate or sodium taurocholate (bile solution)
	Tubes containing 1 ml nutrient broth
	Optochin disks
	Forceps
	Blood agar plate
	Candle jar
	Blood agar plate cultures of pneumococci and other alpha-hemolytic streptococci

Procedures

1. Examine the blood plate cultures of pneumococci and of alpha-hemolytic streptococci for any reliable distinctions in colonial morphology. Make a Gram stain of each organism.
2. Using two tubes of nutrient broth, make a light suspension of pneumococci in each. Repeat, making two suspensions of the other streptococci in nutrient broth.
3. To one tube of each suspended organism add a few drops of the 10% bile solution. Over a 15-minute period, observe all tubes for evidence of clearing of the suspension (lysis of the organisms) and record results for each tube.
4. Mark a blood agar plate with your marking pencil to divide it in half. Streak one side heavily with a loopful of pneumococci, the other side equally with alpha-hemolytic streptococci.
5. Flame your forceps lightly and use them to take up an optochin disk. Place the disk in the center of the area on the blood plate you streaked with pneumococci. Reflame the forceps and place another disk in the middle of the section streaked with alpha-hemolytic streptococci. Press each disk down lightly on the agar with the tip of the forceps, to make certain it is in contact and will not fall off when the plate is inverted (do not press it *through* the agar). Reflame the forceps.

   (*Note:* Optochin is the commercial name for ethylhydrocupreine hydrochloride, a surface reactant impregnated in the disk. Its effect on pneumococcal cell surfaces is similar to that of bile. The disk is often called a "P-disk" because it is used to distinguish susceptible pneumococci from other streptococci that are not lysed by surface reactants.)
6. Invert the plate and place it in a candle jar. Light the candle, replace the lid of the jar (tightly), and wait for the candle flame to burn out. Place the jar in the 35°C incubator for 24 hours. (Any wide-mouthed, screw-cap jar can serve as a candle jar. The candle burning in the closed jar uses up some of the oxygen and increases the carbon dioxide level. At a certain point, the oxygen is not sufficient for the candle to continue burning, and the flame will be extinguished. The atmosphere then remaining within the jar contains the increased carbon dioxide tension and the reduced oxygen tension preferred by many bacterial species, such as pneumococci, when they are first removed from the body and cultured on artificial medium [fig. 19.3].)

Results

1. Record your observations of the colonial and microscopic morphology of pneumococci and other alpha-hemolytic streptococci in the table following step 3 on page 139.
2. Record results of the bile solubility test in the table. Describe here the appearance of each tube at the end of the 15-minute test:

   Pneumococcus suspension with bile _____

   without bile _____

   Alpha-hemolytic *Streptococcus* suspension with bile _____

   without bile _____

Figure 19.3 A closed candle jar containing petri plate cultures. The candle flame has gone out because the remaining oxygen is not sufficient to keep the flame lit. The jar now contains increased carbon dioxide and decreased oxygen, an atmosphere (microaerophilic) preferred by many bacteria.

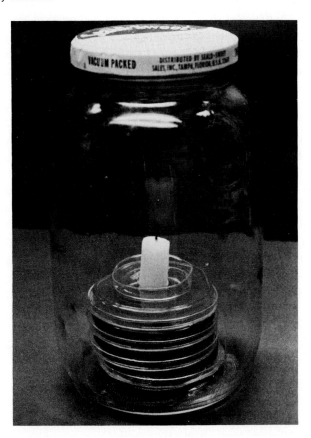

3. Record results of the optochin disk test in the table. Diagram the appearance of the growth on the plate with the disks, indicating your interpretation.

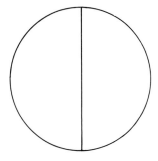

Name of Organism	Colonial Morphology (and Hemolysis)	Microscopic Morphology	Bile Solubility (+ or −)	Optochin Susceptibility (+ or −)
Streptococcus pneumoniae				
Alpha-hemolytic Streptococcus				

EXPERIMENT 19.4 Identification of Enterococci

Enterococci are gram-positive cocci that form chains in culture and that, until recently, were classified in the genus *Streptococcus*. Because they differ in several characteristics, including the composition of their genetic material, they are now classified in a separate genus, *Enterococcus*. As the name implies, enterococci are found primarily in the intestinal tract, although they may be found in the upper respiratory tracts of infants and young children. Their primary role in disease is as the agents of urinary tract infection, infective endocarditis (like the viridans group streptococci), and wound infections, especially those contaminated with intestinal contents. In the laboratory, their colonies resemble somewhat those of group B streptococci. They must be differentiated from this organism because their presence at certain body sites has a different meaning. For example, enterococci isolated from a genital tract specimen of a pregnant woman near term may simply represent contamination from the intestinal tract, whereas isolation of group B streptococci from the same specimen represents a potential hazard for the fetus. In addition, enterococci are more resistant to antimicrobial agents than are streptococci, and the infections they cause must be treated with different drugs. *Enterococcus faecalis* is the most common species isolated from persons with enterococcal infections.

Enterococci previously were known as group D streptococci because they possess a characteristic antigen on their cell wall that reacts in serological tests with group D antibody. Unlike the streptococci, enterococci can grow in a high concentration salt broth (containing 6.5% sodium chloride), are resistant to bile, and hydrolyze a complex carbohydrate, esculin. The last two characteristics are used in a selective and differential medium for enterococci, called bile-esculin agar. The bile inhibits streptococcal but not enterococcal growth. When enterococci hydrolyze the esculin, a black pigment forms in the medium. The pigment results from the reaction of the esculin breakdown products with an iron salt that is also included in the medium. This test often becomes positive within 4 hours so that a rapid identification can be made.

Purpose	To identify enterococci in culture
Materials	6.5% sodium chloride broths
	Plate of bile-esculin agar
	Blood agar plate cultures of *Enterococcus faecalis* and a group B *Streptococcus*

Procedures

1. Examine the blood agar plate culture of the *Enterococcus*. Do the colonies resemble those of the group B *Streptococcus*? Make a Gram stain of the organisms.
2. Inoculate two sodium chloride broths *lightly,* one each with a portion of a colony from each plate. After you inoculate them, the broths should not be turbid; otherwise, you will not be able to determine whether the organism grew during incubation.
3. Incubate the broths for 24 hours at 35°C.
4. Mark the bottom of the bile-esculin plate to divide it in half.
5. Streak the *Enterococcus* across one-half of the bile-esculin agar plate and the group B *Streptococcus* across the other half. Incubate the plate at 35°C and examine it just before you leave the laboratory (don't forget to reincubate) and again after 24 hours.
6. Examine the salt broths for the presence or absence of growth (turbidity). Compare the inoculated, incubated broths with an uninoculated broth tube.
7. Examine the bile-esculin plate and note the color of the medium in each half.

Results

1. For each organism, record results (+ or −) of the esculin hydrolysis reaction (black pigment formation) at the end of the lab session (less than or equal to [≤] 4 hours) and at 24 hours.

    Enterococcus faecalis: ≤4 hours _____

                                            24 hours _____

    group B *Streptococcus:*   ≤4 hours _____

                                            24 hours _____

2. Record your observations in the following table.

| Name of Organism | Colonial Morphology | Microscopic Morphology | Bile-Esculin | | Salt Broth |
			Growth (+ or −)	Pigment (+ or −)	Growth (+ or −)
Enterococcus faecalis					
Group B Streptococcus					

EXPERIMENT 19.5   Streptococci in the Normal Flora

Purpose	To study the normal flora of the throat
Materials	Sheep blood agar plate
	Sterile swab
	Sterile tongue depressor
	Optional:
	Simulated swab from suspected "strep" throat patient
	Kit for detection and confirmation of group A streptococcal antigen from a throat swab

Figure 19.4 Taking a throat culture. The swab should touch *only* the pharyngeal membranes.

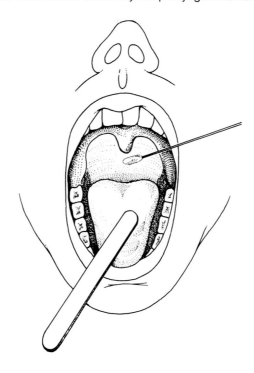

Procedures

1. Figure 19.4 diagrams the correct method for collecting a throat culture. Note that the tongue is held down out of the way and the throat swab is lightly touching the posterior wall of the pharynx.
2. The instructor will demonstrate the method. Observe carefully.
3. Now take a throat culture from your laboratory partner. The "patient" should be positioned in good light so that you can see the back of the throat and the position of the swab as you insert it. *Gently* swab the posterior membranes of the throat, being careful not to touch the swab to any other tissues as you insert or remove it.
4. Inoculate a blood agar plate by rolling the swab over a small area near one edge. Streak the plate with the wire loop, using the streak dilution technique.
5. Discard the swab and tongue depressor in a container of disinfectant.
6. With your flamed loop, make a few stabs in the agar at the area where the swab was rolled. Do not stab through to the bottom of the agar layer. Incubate the plate at 35°C for 24 hours.
7. If the group A streptococcal antigen test kit is available, take a second swab from your "patient" (step 3). Test both your "patient" swab and the simulated swab from the "strep" throat patient following the manufacturer's instructions carefully.

Results

1. If the streptococcal antigen detection test was performed, record the results:

   Your "patient" (+ or −) _____

   "Strep" throat patient (+ or −) _____

Diagnostic Microbiology in Action

Complete the following if the test you used was an EIA test:

Color of the positive test: _____

Color of the negative test: _____

2. Examine the culture plate carefully. How many colonies of different types can you distinguish? Describe each colony type in the following table.
3. Hold the plate against a good light. Do you see any hemolytic colonies? Indicate type of hemolysis shown by each colony recorded in the table.
4. Make a Gram stain of one colony of each type and record results in the table.
5. Enter your tentative identification of each colony in the table and the additional tests needed to complete the identification.

Colony Morphology	Type of Hemolysis	Gram-Stain Reaction	Tentative Identification	Further Tests Needed

6. Did the culture of your "patient's" throat confirm the results of the swab antigen detection test?

Questions

1. Differentiate the microscopic morphology of streptococci and pneumococci as seen by Gram stain.

2. What type of hemolysis is produced by *S. pneumoniae*?

3. How is *S. pneumoniae* distinguished from other streptococci with the same hemolytic properties?

4. What is the quellung reaction?

5. What role does a bacterial capsule play in infection?

6. What kind of culture media and atmospheric and incubation conditions are best for cultivating streptococci?

7. Is blood agar a differential medium? Why?

8. What is the function of a candle jar?

9. Describe alpha-hemolytic, beta-hemolytic, and nonhemolytic streptococci.

10. What type of hemolysis is displayed by streptococci that are most pathogenic for human beings?

_____

To what serological group do these usually belong? _____

How can they be identified as belonging to this group without doing a serological test? Explain.

11. Describe the principle of the latex agglutination test.

12. Name at least three bacterial species found among the normal flora of the throat.

13. Is the normal flora of the upper respiratory tract harmful to the human host? If so, explain.

14. Is the normal flora beneficial to the host? If so, explain.

15. In collecting a throat culture, why is it important not to touch the swab to other surfaces in the mouth?

16. What specimens are of value in making a laboratory diagnosis of bacterial pneumonia? Why? Explain the difference between saliva and sputum.

17. Would a direct Gram stain of a sputum specimen be of any immediate value to the physician in choosing treatment for a patient with pneumonia? Explain.

18. Does antimicrobial therapy have any effect on the body's normal flora? Explain.

EXERCISE 20   Staphylococci

Reference: Morello, Mizer, Wilson, and Granato, Microbiology in Patient Care, 5th edition, 1994. Chapters 12, 19.

Staphylococci are ubiquitous in our environment and in the normal flora of our bodies. They are particularly numerous on skin and in the upper respiratory tract, including the anterior nares as well as pharyngeal surfaces. Some are also associated with human infectious diseases.

Staphylococci are gram-positive cocci, characteristically arranged in irregular clusters like grapes (see colorplate 1). They are hardy, facultatively aerobic organisms that grow well on most nutrient media. There are three principal species: *Staphylococcus epidermidis, Staphylococcus saprophyticus,* and *Staphylococcus aureus. S. epidermidis,* as its name implies, is the most frequent inhabitant of human surface tissues, including mucous membranes. It is not usually pathogenic, but it may cause serious infections if it has an unusual opportunity for entry, as in cardiac surgery or in patients with indwelling intravenous catheters who usually have low resistance. *S. saprophyticus* has been implicated in acute urinary tract infections in young women approximately 16 to 25 years of age. It has not been found among the normal flora and is not yet known to cause other types of infection. It is included in this exercise for completeness. Like *S. epidermidis, S. aureus* is often found among the normal flora of healthy persons, but in addition, most staphylococcal disease is caused by strains of this species.

S. aureus strains produce a number of toxins and enzymes that can exert harmful effects on the cells of the infected host. Their *hemolysins* can destroy red blood cells. The enzyme *coagulase* coagulates plasma, but its exact role in staphylococcal infection is not yet known. *Leukocidin* is a staphylococcal toxin that destroys leukocytes. *Hyaluronidase* is an enzyme that acts on a substrate that is a structural component of connective tissue. Its activity in a local area of infection breaks down the tissue and permits the staphylococci to penetrate more deeply; hence, it is called "spreading factor." (Some streptococci also produce hyaluronidase.) *Staphylokinase* can dissolve fibrin clots, thus enhancing the invasiveness of organisms that would otherwise be walled off by the body's fibrinous reactions. An *enterotoxin* is elaborated by some strains of *S. aureus.* If these are multiplying in contaminated food, the enterotoxin they produce can be responsible for severe gastroenteritis or staphylococcal food poisoning. Some strains produce toxic shock syndrome (TSS) by elaborating a toxin referred to as TSST-1. This disease is seen primarily in menstruating women who use highly absorbent tampons. *S. aureus* colonizing the vaginal tract multiplies there and releases TSST-1 causing a variety of symptoms including shock and a rash. TSS has also been documented in children, men, and nonmenstruating women who have a focus of infection at nongenital sites. Strains of *S. epidermidis* and *S. saprophyticus* do not produce these toxic substances.

Common skin infections caused by *S. aureus* include pimples, furuncles (boils), carbuncles, and impetigo. Serious systemic (deep tissue) infections that result from *S. aureus* invasion include pneumonia, pyelonephritis, osteomyelitis, meningitis, and endocarditis. Infection by staphylococci of the membranes of the upper respiratory tract, its lymphatic tissue, or its extensions into sinuses and the eustachian canal may result in tonsillitis, sinusitis, or otitis media.

EXPERIMENT 20.1   Isolation and Identification of Staphylococci

The laboratory diagnosis of staphylococcal disease is made by identifying the organism (usually *S. aureus*) in a clinical specimen representing the site of infection (pus from a skin lesion, sputum when pneumonia is suspected, urine, spinal fluid, or blood). It should be remembered that either *S. aureus* or *S. epidermidis* may be harmlessly present on superficial tissues. Special care must be taken not to permit contamination of the specimen with normal flora, if this is possible, and laboratory results must be interpreted in the light of the patient's clinical symptoms. The principal features by which staphylococci are recognized and distinguished in the laboratory include their microscopic morphology, colonial appearance on blood agar (especially hemolytic activity), coagulase activity (see colorplate 21), reaction to the carbohydrate mannitol, and susceptibility to the antimicrobial agent novobiocin. The species are indistinguishable microscopically.

On blood agar, *S. aureus* usually displays a pigment having a light to golden yellow color (hence, its name), whereas *S. epidermidis* has a white pigment and *S. saprophyticus* either a bright yellow or white pigment. However, pigmentation is not a fully reliable characteristic. On blood agar, *S. aureus* is usually, but not always, beta-hemolytic; *S. epidermidis* and *S. saprophyticus* are almost always nonhemolytic. *S. aureus* is, by definition, coagulase positive; *S. epidermidis* and *S. saprophyticus* are coagulase negative. Other *Staphylococcus* species that are found on skin but seldom cause disease are also coagulase negative. As a group, these species, along with *S. epidermidis* and *S. saprophyticus* are referred to as *coagulase-negative staphylococci*. *S. aureus* is further distinguished by its ability to ferment mannitol, and *S. saprophyticus* by its resistance to low concentrations of novobiocin.

Since specimens from the mucous membranes or skin may contain a mixed normal flora as well as the pathogenic staphylococci being sought, the use of a selective, differential medium in the primary isolation battery can be very helpful (see Table 16.1). Mannitol salt agar is such a medium. It contains a high concentration of salt that inhibits gram-positive cocci other than staphylococci and many other organisms as well. It also contains mannitol and an indicator to differentiate *S. aureus* strains from coagulase-negative staphylococci growing on it. A blood agar plate is also essential for demonstrating hemolytic organisms. Since some streptococci, as well as many strains of *S. aureus,* are beta-hemolytic, they can be distinguished promptly. Aside from microscopic morphology, the simplest, most rapid distinction can be made with the catalase test, for all streptococci are catalase negative, whereas all staphylococci are catalase positive.

Staphylococcus aureus is carried by a large segment of the population as a member of the normal flora. It is a threat primarily to individuals with lowered resistance, particularly to patients in hospitals. In the hospital, *S. aureus* is a major cause of nosocomial infections transmitted from hospital personnel or the environment. The problem is compounded by the fact that many "hospital" strains of staphylococci are resistant to the useful antimicrobial agents. All personnel involved in patient care should be knowledgeable of transmission routes and carefully follow the technical routines designed to prevent nosocomial infection. In the experiments that follow, you will be seeing and handling staphylococcal cultures. Apply your knowledge of aseptic technique and make certain that you do not carry staphylococci out of the laboratory as new additions to the flora of your hands or clothes. Keep your hands scrupulously clean. If you have any minor cuts or scratches or other injury to your hands, they should be protected. While in the laboratory, keep your hands (pencils, too) away from your mouth and face.

Purpose	To isolate and identify staphylococci from broth cultures
Materials	Blood agar plate (BAP)
	Mannitol salt agar plate (MSA)
	Tubed plasma (0.5-ml aliquots)
	Novobiocin disks (5 μg)
	Sterile 1.0-ml pipettes
	Pipette bulb or other aspiration device
	Forceps
	Beaker containing 70% alcohol
	24-hour broth cultures of *Staphylococcus epidermidis, Staphylococcus aureus,*
	Staphylococcus saprophyticus, and *Escherichia coli*

Procedures

1. With your marking pencil, divide the bottom of a BAP and an MSA plate into four segments each.
2. Using the grown broth cultures, inoculate one section of each plate with *S. aureus,* one with *S. epidermidis,* one with *S. saprophyticus,* and one with *E. coli.* Streak each section carefully, remaining within the assigned space.
3. Dip the tips of the forceps in 70% alcohol, flame rapidly, and allow to cool.
4. Pick up a novobiocin disk, place it in the center of one of the streaked areas of the BAP and press it gently onto the agar with the forcep tips.

5. Repeat steps 3 and 4 for the remaining three organisms on the streaked BAP.
6. Place the plates in the 35°C incubator for 24 hours.
7. Perform a coagulase test on each of the three *Staphylococcus* broth cultures as follows:
   a. Using a sterile pipette, measure 0.1 ml of the *S. epidermidis* broth culture with the aspiration device. Transfer this inoculum to a tube of plasma. Discard the pipette in disinfectant. Label the tube.
   b. Inoculate a second and third tube of plasma with 0.1 ml of the *S. aureus* and *S. saprophyticus* broth cultures, respectively, as in step 7a.
   c. Place all inoculated plasma tubes in the 35°C incubator. After 30 minutes, remove and examine them (close the incubator door while you read them). Hold the tubes in a semihorizontal position to see whether the plasma in the tube is beginning to clot into a solid mass. If so, make a record of the tube showing coagulase activity. Return unclotted tubes to the incubator.
   d. Repeat procedure 7c every 30 minutes for 4 hours, if necessary.
8. After 24 hours of incubation of the plate cultures prepared in procedures 1 and 2, examine and record colonial morphology. Make Gram stains of each culture on the BAP and record microscopic morphology. Measure and record the diameter of the zone of inhibition around the novobiocin disks. A zone size greater than 12 mm in diameter is considered susceptible.

Results

1. Table of plate culture results:

Name of Organism	Colonial Morphology on BAP	Microscopic Morphology (BAP)	Appearance on MSA	Microscopic Morphology (MSA)	Novobiocin Zone Diameter
S. epidermidis					
S. aureus					
S. saprophyticus					
E. coli					X

2. Results of identification tests:

Name of Organism	Coagulase (+ or −)	Time Required to Clot Plasma	Appearance of Plasma After 4 hr.	Mannitol* (+ or −)	Novobiocin* (S or R)
S. epidermidis					
S. aureus					
S. saprophyticus					

*Your interpretation of results in 1 above.

EXPERIMENT 20.2   Staphylococci in the Normal Flora

Purpose	To isolate and identify staphylococci in cultures of the nose and hands
Materials	Blood agar plates (BAP) Mannitol salt agar plates (MSA) Sterile swabs Dropping bottle containing hydrogen peroxide Tubed plasma (0.5-ml aliquots)

Procedures

1. Take a culture of your own nose by swabbing the membrane of one of your anterior nares with a sterile swab.
2. Inoculate the nasal swab across the top quarter of a blood agar and a mannitol salt agar plate. Streak across the remainder of each plate for isolation of colonies. Discard the swab in disinfectant.
3. Take a culture from the palm of your left hand by swabbing across it. Inoculate a blood agar and a mannitol salt agar plate and streak for isolation of colonies.
4. Sterilize your inoculating loop and moisten it in sterile saline. Run the moistened loop under one of your fingernails, picking up some debris if possible. Inoculate a blood agar and a mannitol salt agar plate and streak out.
5. Incubate all plates at 35°C for 24 hours.
6. Examine the plates and make Gram stains of different colony types on both the blood and mannitol plates. Perform a catalase test on the different colony types on both blood and mannitol plates by placing a drop of hydrogen peroxide on a clean glass slide and emulsifying a loopful of a colony in the drop. Observe for bubble formation. Perform a coagulase test on a colony of mannitol-positive staphylococci, if present, using your loop to pick it from an MSA plate and emulsify it directly in 0.5 ml of plasma (continue as in Exp. 20.1 steps 7c and d).
7. Record your observations in the following table.

Results

Colony Morphology on Blood Agar Plate	Microscopic Morphology (BAP)	Catalase (+ or −) (BAP)	Appearance on Mannitol Salt Agar	Microscopic Morphology (MSA)	Catalase (+ or −) (MSA)	Coagulase (+ or −) (Man +)

In the last column, indicate the tentative identification you would make of each colony described in the table.

Questions

1. Differentiate the microscopic morphology of staphylococci and streptococci as seen by Gram stain.

2. What is coagulase?

3. What properties of *S. aureus* distinguish it from *S. epidermidis* and *S. saprophyticus*?

4. How is *S. saprophyticus* distinguished from *S. epidermidis*?

5. From what specimen type would *S. saprophyticus* most likely be isolated?

6. What is a nosocomial infection? Who acquires it? Why?

7. Why are staphylococcal infections frequent among hospital patients?

8. Discuss the role played by *S. aureus* in human infectious diseases.

EXERCISE 21 *Klebsiella* and *Haemophilus*

Reference: Morello, Mizer, Wilson, and Granato, Microbiology in Patient Care, *5th edition, 1994.*
Chapters 12, 15.

EXPERIMENT **21.1** *Klebsiella*

Klebsiella pneumoniae is also sometimes associated with pneumonia. It is a gram-negative, nonmotile bacillus (see colorplate 5) often found among the enteric bacilli normally inhabiting the intestinal tract. When it finds an opportunity to invade the lungs (or other soft tissues), it can cause infection. Like the pneumococcus, pathogenic strains of *K. pneumoniae* possess a slimy, protective capsule (larger and more pronounced than most bacterial capsules; see colorplate 12).

Laboratory diagnosis of *Klebsiella* pneumonia is made by identifying the organism in cultures of sputum or pleural fluid. *K. pneumoniae* grows well aerobically on a variety of culture media. If a differential lactose agar plate such as EMB is included in the primary isolation battery, this organism produces large, mucoid colonies that ferment the lactose. A few key biochemical tests then serve to identify the isolated organism (see also Exercise 24). The quellung reaction is sometimes used to demonstrate the capsule and to distinguish serological types of *Klebsiella*.

Purpose	To identify *K. pneumoniae* in culture
Materials	Blood agar plate
	EMB plate
	Lactose phenol red broth with Durham tube
	Glucose phenol red broth with Durham tube
	Tube of SIM medium
	Xylene
	Kovac's reagent
	Agar slant culture of *K. pneumoniae*

Procedures

1. Make a Gram stain of the culture of *K. pneumoniae* and record results.
2. Inoculate an EMB and a blood agar plate with the culture. Streak for isolation of colonies.
3. Inoculate one tube each of glucose and lactose phenol red broth and SIM tubed agar (stab the latter to one-fourth the depth of the medium).
4. Incubate all cultures at 35°C for 24 hours.
5. Examine colonial morphology on the plated cultures. Record your observations in the Results table.
6. Examine the carbohydrate broths for evidence of fermentation and record results in the table.
7. Examine the SIM tube for evidence of motility and H_2S production.
8. Test the SIM culture for evidence of indole production.

Results

Organism	Appearance on EMB plate	Appearance on Blood Plate	Microscopic Morphology	Indole (+ or −)	Motility (+ or −)	H₂S (+ or −)
Klebsiella pneumoniae						
Carbohydrate fermentation:		Acid	Acid + gas	Alkaline	Negative	
Lactose:						
Glucose:						

EXPERIMENT 21.2   *Haemophilus*

The genus *Haemophilus* contains a number of species of fastidious, gram-negative bacilli. Most of these are found as normal flora on the membranes of the upper respiratory tract. *Haemophilus* species can cause infections in a variety of sites in the upper respiratory tract and elsewhere in the body. Laboratory diagnosis is made by identifying these organisms in clinical specimens appropriately representing the area of infection (throat swab, sinus drainage, sputum, conjunctival swab, spinal fluid, blood, or other). A direct smear of the specimen may be useful, particularly for spinal fluid or an exudate from the eye, in providing rapid, presumptive information. (Smears of material from the upper respiratory tract, with its mixed flora, may have little value unless the organisms are present in large numbers.) Latex or coagglutination antibody tests can also be performed directly with certain patient body fluids to detect *Haemophilus* antigen (see Exp. 19.1). Most serious *Haemophilus* disease is caused by the species *influenzae,* and the serogroup b.

These fastidious *Haemophilus* organisms require specially enriched culture media and microaerophilic incubation conditions. In addition to blood agar plates, "chocolate" agar is commonly used for primary isolation of *Haemophilus* from clinical specimens. This medium contains hemoglobin derived from bovine red blood cells as well as other enrichment growth factors. Because the hemoglobin is dark brown, the agar in the plate has the appearance of chocolate.

Two special growth factors, called X and V, are required by some *Haemophilus* species. Some require one but not the other. The X factor is *hemin,* a heat-stable derivative of hemoglobin (supplied in chocolate agar). The V factor is a heat-labile coenzyme (nicotinamide adenine dinucleotide or NAD), essential in the metabolism of some species that lack it. Yeast extracts contain V factor and are one of the most convenient supplements of chocolate agar or other media used for *Haemophilus.* Organisms other than yeasts elaborate V factor. Staphylococci, for example, when growing on an agar plate secrete NAD into the surrounding medium. *Haemophilus* species that need V factor may grow in the zone immediately around the staphylococci but not elsewhere on the plate. This growth of the dependent organism is described as "satellitism" (see colorplate 22). X and V factors can also be impregnated in filter-paper disks pressed on the surface of media otherwise deficient in these factors. In this experiment the identification of *Haemophilus* by its growth characteristics and requirements will be illustrated.

Purpose	To identify *Haemophilus* species in culture
Materials	Sheep blood agar plate
	Chocolate agar plate
	Nutrient agar plate
	X and V disks
	Forceps
	Candle jar
	Chocolate agar plate cultures of *Haemophilus influenzae* and *Haemophilus parainfluenzae*
	Demonstration blood agar and nutrient agar plates showing satellitism

Procedures

1. Make a Gram stain of each species of *Haemophilus*.
2. Pencil-divide a sheep blood plate and a chocolate agar plate in half. Inoculate *H. influenzae* on one side of each plate and streak for isolation within this half. Repeat with *H. parainfluenzae* on the other half of each plate. Incubate these plates in a candle jar at 35°C for 24 hours.
3. Repeat step 2 using the nutrient agar plate, but inoculate each strain heavily and streak for confluent growth within its half of the plate. Now, using flamed, cooled forceps, place an X and a V disk on the agar surface streaked with *H. influenzae* and repeat on the *H. parainfluenzae* side. The two disks on each side should be placed not more than 1 inch apart, and centered in the area streaked (see diagram under Results 3). Incubate this plate in a candle jar at 35°C for 24 hours.
4. Examine the demonstration plates. *H. influenzae* has been streaked heavily on one-half of each plate, *H. parainfluenzae* on the other half. An inoculum of a *Staphylococcus* culture was made in one area in the center of each streaked portion. Describe your observations and indicate your interpretation of the appearance of the blood and nutrient agar plates under Results 4.

Results

1. Describe the microscopic morphology of the two *Haemophilus* species you Gram stained, indicating any distinctions you observed between them.

2. Describe the colonial morphology of each *Haemophilus* species:

Organism	Chocolate Agar	Blood Agar

How do you interpret growth versus no growth on these plates?

3. Diagram the appearance of the growth of each *Haemophilus* species on the nutrient agar plate with X and V disks and interpret.

H. influenzae

Interpretation:

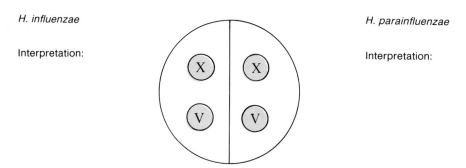

H. parainfluenzae

Interpretation:

4. Diagram the appearance of the demonstration plates and interpret.

H. influenzae

Interpretation:

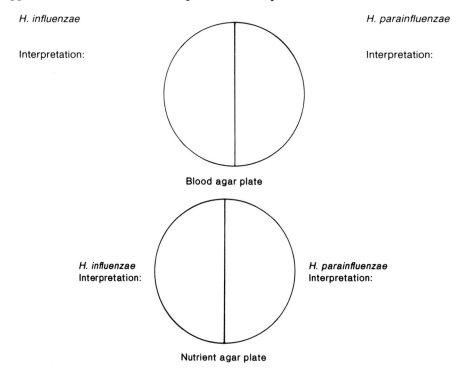

H. parainfluenzae

Interpretation:

Blood agar plate

H. influenzae
Interpretation:

H. parainfluenzae
Interpretation:

Nutrient agar plate

Questions

1. Can you distinguish *Streptococcus pneumoniae* from *Klebsiella pneumoniae* by Gram stain? Explain. (Refer to your notes for Experiment 19.3.)

2. Describe the differences you observed in the colonial appearance of *S. pneumoniae* (Experiment 19.3) and *K. pneumoniae* on blood agar.

3. Which of these organisms is considered fastidious? Why?

4. Why is EMB useful in the primary isolation of *K. pneumoniae*?

5. What is chocolate agar?

6. Define X and V factors.

7. What is the clinical significance of a laboratory report of *S. pneumoniae* or *K. pneumoniae* identified in a sputum culture?

8. Name three species of *Haemophilus* and indicate the types of infection with which each may be associated.

9. What is the satellite phenomenon?

10. What is the incidence of *Haemophilus influenzae* as an agent of meningitis in infants and children under 3 years of age? In adults?

11. Why is a direct smear of spinal fluid essential when bacterial meningitis is suspected?

EXERCISE 22 Corynebacteria and *Bordetella*

Reference: Morello, Mizer, Wilson, and Granato, Microbiology in Patient Care, 5th edition, 1994. Chapter 12.

EXPERIMENT 22.1   Corynebacteria

The genus *Corynebacterium* is comprised of many species, but *Corynebacterium diphtheriae* has the most important pathogenic properties. *C. diphtheriae* is the agent of diphtheria, a serious throat infection and a systemic, toxic disease. If they have an opportunity to colonize in the throat, virulent strains of this organism not only damage the local tissue (causing formation of a *pseudomembrane*), but they produce a powerful *exotoxin* that disseminates through the body from the site of its production in the upper respiratory tract. When this toxin reaches the cells of the myocardium, adrenal cortex, or other vital organs, it has very damaging effects. The systemic effect of toxin is the primary cause of death in those patients with diphtheria who are not promptly recognized and treated. The disease is controlled by maintaining active immunization with diphtheria *toxoid* (purified toxin treated so that it is no longer toxic but remains immunogenic).

Early clinical and laboratory recognition of diphtheria infection developing in the throat is vital, for prompt treatment with antitoxin (antibody that neutralizes the toxin) and an appropriate antimicrobial agent can assure the patient's recovery. In the laboratory, the microbiologist must distinguish *C. diphtheriae* from other corynebacteria that may be present in a smear or culture of the throat exudate as harmless members of the normal flora. This must be done as rapidly as possible, for the laboratory report is an essential basis for clinical decisions. In patients with decreased immune functions (referred to as *immunocompromised* patients), these other corynebacteria may cause disease by invading the weakened host to produce bacteremia and pneumonia.

Corynebacteria are gram-positive, nonmotile, nonsporing bacilli, as ubiquitous as staphylococci in their distribution on our bodies and in the environment. Nonpathogenic species are often called *diphtheroids* because they resemble *C. diphtheriae* in microscopic morphology. These rods often contain granules that stain irregularly (they are said to be *metachromatic*) and give the organisms a beaded or clubbed appearance. Pairs or small groups characteristically fall into patterns that look like Chinese letters, or like Vs and Ys. Usually, *C. diphtheriae* is longer, thinner, and more beaded in appearance than diphtheroids, which are generally short and thick by comparison. This differentiation can be very difficult to make in examining a stained throat smear and cannot be relied on for accurate diagnosis.

In culture, corynebacteria are not highly fastidious. They grow well aerobically on nutrient media. When diphtheria is suspected, the primary isolation media used for throat swabs include those that are selective and differential for *C. diphtheriae* and also blood agar. Loeffler's serum medium is commonly used for direct inoculation and transport of the swab to the laboratory. This is a firm coagulated serum medium containing nutrient broth, prepared as a tubed slant. It is somewhat selective in that it is not sufficiently enriched for many of the fastidious organisms of the throat flora, and therefore corynebacteria growing on it are not greatly crowded by many other organisms. Some others (especially staphylococci), however, can be expected to grow. Serum or blood agar to which potassium tellurite has been added constitutes a good selective and differential medium for primary isolation of *C. diphtheriae*. The tellurite not only suppresses many other throat flora, but it is metabolized by *C. diphtheriae* with resulting blackening of its colonial growth. Thus the organism is differentiated from others that can grow on the agar medium. The use of blood agar in the initial battery assures the recovery of corynebacteria, as well as other pathogenic bacterial species that might be present, and differentiates those that are hemolytic.

The biochemical differentiation of *C. diphtheriae* from other corynebacteria is based on carbohydrate fermentations. Demonstration of toxin production is essential in reporting identification of a strain of *C. diphtheriae,* for not all strains are toxigenic. Tests for virulence, that is, toxigenicity, are made either in experimental animals (rabbits or guinea pigs) or by an in vitro method (Elek test). In the Elek test, antitoxin strips are placed on agar plates to detect toxin produced by strains of *C. diphtheriae* growing on the medium. Although virulence tests are not included in this exercise, you should familiarize yourself with these procedures and their purpose by reading the reference material cited for the exercise.

Purpose	To identify corynebacteria in smears and cultures
Materials	Blood agar plate
	Blood tellurite plate
	Tubed phenol red glucose broth
	Tubed phenol red maltose broth
	Tubed phenol red sucrose broth
	Prepared Gram-stained smears of *C. diphtheriae*
	Loeffler's slant cultures of *Corynebacterium xerosis* and *Corynebacterium pseudodiphtheriticum*
	Nutrient agar slant culture of *Escherichia coli*

Procedures

1. Prepare a Gram stain and a methylene blue stain (see Exercise 4) from either one of the *Corynebacterium* cultures. Read and compare these with the Gram-stained smear of *C. diphtheriae,* recording your observations under Results.
2. Inoculate a blood agar plate with either one of the *Corynebacterium* cultures. Streak for isolation.
3. Divide the blood tellurite plate into two parts with your marker. Inoculate one side of the plate with a *Corynebacterium* species, the other side with *E. coli*.
4. Inoculate the *C. xerosis* culture into each of the three carbohydrate broths. Repeat with the culture of *C. pseudodiphtheriticum.*
5. Incubate all plate and tube cultures at 35°C for 24 hours.
6. Examine your cultures and record your observations.

Results

1. Illustrate the microscopic morphology of corynebacteria:

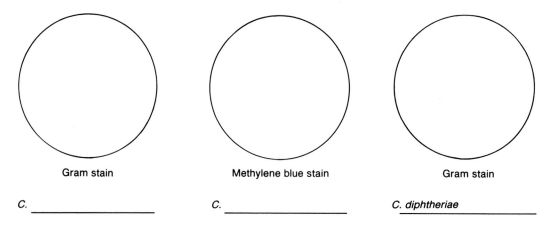

Gram stain	Methylene blue stain	Gram stain
C. _____	C. _____	*C. diphtheriae* _____

2. Describe the appearance of a *Corynebacterium* species on blood agar.

3. Describe the appearance of *E. coli* and of a *Corynebacterium* species on blood tellurite agar.

4. Complete the following table:

Name of Organism	Glucose	Maltose	Sucrose
C. xerosis			
C. pseudodiphtheriticum			
C. diphtheriae	+	+	−

EXPERIMENT 22.2 *Bordetella*

Bordetella pertussis is the etiologic agent of whooping cough. This very fastidious organism grows best on special media. The two most common are Bordet-Gengou (BG) agar, which is enriched with glycerin, potato, and 30% defibrinated sheep blood, and Regan-Lowe (RL) agar, which consists of charcoal agar, defibrinated horse blood, and an antimicrobial agent to inhibit growth of normal respiratory flora. The charcoal is present to adsorb toxic substances that might be present in the agar. Visible colonies are produced only after three to five days incubation in a microaerophilic atmosphere. On BG medium, the colonies are raised, rounded, and glistening (resembling mercury droplets or a bisected pearl), and usually have a hazy zone of hemolysis. On RL medium, the colonies are round, domed, shiny, and may run together slightly.

   B. pertussis is a gram-negative bacillus resembling *Haemophilus* species, with which it was once classified. When whooping cough is suspected, the best specimen for laboratory diagnosis is a nasopharyngeal swab, but throat swabs may be used in addition.

Purpose	To observe *Bordetella pertussis* in demonstration and to examine a throat culture on Bordet-Gengou (BG) and Regan-Lowe (RL) media
Materials	Prepared Gram stains of *B. pertussis* Projection slides, if available Bordet-Gengou and Regan-Lowe agar plates

Procedures

1. Examine the prepared Gram stains and record your observations.
2. Observe colonial morphology as demonstrated.
3. Collect a throat specimen as in Experiment 19.5 and inoculate the Bordet-Gengou and Regan-Lowe plates. Incubate the plates at 35°C in a candle jar for 24 hours.

Results

1. Describe the microscopic morphology of *B. pertussis*.

2. Describe your observations of demonstration material.

3. Describe the appearance of your Bordet-Gengou and Regan-Lowe throat culture plates.

   What is the total number of colonies? BG _____ RL _____

   How many colony types can be distinguished? BG _____ RL _____

   How does the flora compare with that of your throat culture in Experiment 19.5?

Questions

1. Name the etiologic agent of diphtheria and describe the media used to isolate it from a clinical specimen.

2. How can a diphtheroid be distinguished from the agent of diphtheria?

3. What is a virulence test and how is it performed?

4. Can diphtheria be transmitted directly via the respiratory route? If so, how?

5. How is diphtheria prevented?

6. Why is early laboratory diagnosis of diphtheria important?

7. What is the etiologic agent of whooping cough and what media are used to isolate it?

8. What is the preferred specimen for diagnosing whooping cough?

9. How can transmission of respiratory infections be prevented?

10. Complete the following chart.

BACTERIA ASSOCIATED WITH THE RESPIRATORY TRACT AND WITH DISEASE

Etiologic Agent	Disease	Specimens for Lab Diagnosis	Microscopic Morphology and Gram-Stain Reaction	Hemolysis (Type)	Key Tests for Lab Identification	Normal Habitat
Beta-hemolytic streptococci group A						
Alpha-hemolytic streptococci						
S. pneumoniae						
E. faecalis						
S. epidermidis						
S. aureus						
C. diphtheriae						
Diphtheroids						
H. influenzae						
H. haemolyticus						
B. pertussis						

Diagnostic Microbiology in Action

EXERCISE 23 Clinical Specimens from the Respiratory Tract

*Reference: Morello, Mizer, Wilson, and Granato, Microbiology in Patient Care, 5th edition, 1994.
Chapter 12.*

Now that you have had some experience with the normal flora and the most common bacterial pathogens of the respiratory tract, you will have an opportunity to apply what you have learned to the laboratory diagnosis of respiratory infections. In the following experiments you will prepare cultures of a throat swab and a sputum specimen, each simulating material that might be obtained from a sick patient. These cultures should be examined with particular attention to the "physician's" stated tentative diagnosis. Significant organisms that may be isolated must be identified and reported. If organisms that you consider to be part of the normal flora are isolated, report as "normal flora."

In the final experiment of this exercise, you will set up an antimicrobial susceptibility test on an organism isolated from one of the clinical specimens previously cultured, and prepare a report for the "physician" of the results.

EXPERIMENT 23.1 Laboratory Diagnosis of a Sore Throat

Purpose	To identify bacterial species in a simulated clinical throat culture as quickly as possible
Materials	*Swab in a tube of broth,* accompanied by a laboratory request for culture
	Patient's name: Mary Peters
	Age: 6 years
	Physician: Dr. M. Selby
	Tentative clinical diagnosis: "Strep sore throat"
	Blood agar plate (BAP)
	Mannitol salt agar plate (MSA)
	Dropping bottle containing hydrogen peroxide
	Tubed plasma (0.5-ml aliquots)
	Tubed nutrient broth (0.5-ml aliquots)
	Sterile 1.0-ml pipettes
	Pipette bulb or other aspiration device

Procedures

1. Make a Gram stain of the simulated throat culture. Record results and place the information in an accessible place pending a telephone call from the "physician."
2. Using the swab in the "specimen" tube, inoculate a blood agar plate and a mannitol plate. Streak each for isolation of colonies. Incubate both plates at 35°C for 24 hours.
3. When the "physician" calls, give him or her specific information about your microscopic interpretation of the Gram-stained smear from the specimen.
4. After the plates have incubated, examine each carefully. Record colonial morphology, and make Gram stains of different colony types on each medium.
5. Apply the catalase test to different colony types on each medium.
6. Apply the coagulase test to any colony on either plate that appears to be a *Staphylococcus*. Do this by emulsifying the colony in 0.5 ml of plasma, using your loop to pick up a portion of the colony and make the suspension. Incubate the inoculated plasma tubes and read at intervals through a 30-minute to 4-hour period. Record.
7. Prepare a final report for the "physician."

Results

1. Initial report of the findings on Gram stain of a direct smear:

2. Final laboratory report to "physician":

MICROBIOLOGY LABORATORY REPORT
Patient's Name: _____
Sex: _____ Age: _____ Date: _____
Tentative Diagnosis: _____
Laboratory Findings:
Direct Smear Report: _____
Culture Result: _____
SIGNATURE: _____ Date Rec'd: _____ Reported: _____
LABORATORY NAME: _____
_____
PHYSICIAN'S NAME: _____

3. Laboratory file information:

Culture No.   Patient's Name: Physician:

Specimen: Date Received: Date Reported:

Name of Organism	Gram Stain and Morphology	Hemolysis	Mannitol	Catalase	Coagulase

Final Report: Signature:

EXPERIMENT **23.2** **Laboratory Diagnosis of Bacterial Pneumonia**

Purpose	To identify bacterial species in a simulated sputum as quickly as possible
Materials	*Simulated sputum in a screw-cap container,* accompanied by a laboratory request for culture

      Patient's name: Richard Wilson
      Age: 72 years
      Physician's name: Dr. F. Smythe
      Tentative diagnosis: Bronchial pneumonia
    Blood agar plate (BAP)
    Mannitol salt agar plate (MSA)
    Eosin methylene blue plate (EMB)
    Media for identification to be selected by student, as indicated by growth on isolation
      plates

Procedures

1. Make a Gram stain of the simulated sputum. Record results and place the information in an accessible place pending a telephone call from the "physician."
2. Using a wire loop, inoculate the specimen on a BAP, MSA, and EMB plate. Incubate all plates at 35°C for 24 hours.
3. When the "physician" calls, give him or her specific information about your microscopic findings and interpretation of the Gram stain of the direct smear from the specimen.
4. After the plates have incubated, examine each carefully. Record colonial morphology and make Gram stains of different colony types on each medium.
5. Select appropriate media and materials from available stock supplies to confirm your tentative identification of isolated colonies. Perform appropriate procedures; incubate subcultures as indicated.
6. Record your final results and prepare a report for the "physician."

Results

1. Initial report of the findings on Gram stain of a direct smear:

2. Final laboratory report to "physician":

MICROBIOLOGY LABORATORY REPORT

Patient's Name: _____

Sex: _____ Age: _____ Date: _____

Tentative Diagnosis: _____

Laboratory Findings:

Direct Smear Report: _____

Culture Result: _____

SIGNATURE: _____ Date Rec'd: _____ Reported: _____

LABORATORY NAME: _____

_____

PHYSICIAN'S NAME: _____

---

3. Laboratory file information:

Culture No.	Patient's Name:		Physician:		
Specimen:	Date Received:			Date Reported:	
Name of Organism	Gram	*	*	*	*
Final Report:			Signature:		

*Fill in appropriate test.

EXPERIMENT **23.3**   **Antimicrobial Susceptibility Test of an Isolate from a Clinical Specimen**

Purpose	To determine the antimicrobial susceptibility pattern of an organism isolated from a clinical specimen (in Exp. 23.1 or 23.2)
Materials	Nutrient agar plates (Mueller-Hinton if available) Antimicrobial disks Sterile swabs Forceps Beaker containing 70% alcohol Blood agar plate with pure culture of isolate Tube of nutrient broth (5.0 ml) McFarland No. 0.5 turbidity standard

Procedures

1. Using a sterile swab, take some of the growth of a pure culture you isolated from the clinical specimen in Experiment 23.1 or 23.2, and emulsify it in 5.0 ml of nutrient broth until the turbidity is equivalent to the McFarland 0.5 standard. Discard the swab.
2. Take another sterile swab, dip it in the broth suspension, drain off excess fluid against the inner wall of the tube.
3. Inoculate an agar plate as described in Experiment 15.1.
4. Follow procedures 4 through 7 of Experiment 15.1.
5. Incubate the agar plate at 35°C for 24 hours.
6. Examine plates and record results for each antimicrobial disk as S (susceptible), MS (moderately susceptible), I (intermediate), or R (resistant).
7. Prepare a report for the "physician."

Results

Record results:

```
┌──────────────────────────────────────────────────────────────────────┐
│                    MICROBIOLOGY LABORATORY REPORT                      │
│                                                                        │
│  Patient's Name _____   │
│                                                                        │
│  Sex: _____ Age: _____ Date: _____    │
│                                                                        │
│  Tentative Diagnosis: _____   │
│                                                                        │
│                     Antimicrobial Susceptibility Report                │
│                                                                        │
│  Name of Organism: _____   │
│                                                                        │
│  Source: _____   │
└──────────────────────────────────────────────────────────────────────┘
```

Antimicrobial Agent	S	MS	I	R	Antimicrobial Agent	S	MS	I	R

SIGNATURE: _____ Date Rec'd: _____ Reported: _____

LABORATORY NAME: _____

_____

PHYSICIAN'S NAME: _____

Questions

1. Is a Gram stain of a throat swab useful for making a rapid, presumptive diagnosis of:
   a. Strep sore throat?

   b. Diphtheria?

2. Is a Gram stain of a sputum specimen useful in making a rapid, presumptive diagnosis of pneumonia?

3. Why should sputum specimens be submitted to the laboratory in screw-cap containers?

4. What is the clinical significance of staphylococci isolated from throat cultures?

5. What is the clinical significance of beta-hemolytic streptococci isolated from throat cultures?

6. In a Gram stain of a sputum specimen, which type of body cell provides an indication that the specimen represents material from an active infection? Why?

7. Should an antimicrobial susceptibility test be performed on every bacterium isolated from a clinical specimen?

8. Why are certain antimicrobial agents tested with either gram-positive or gram-negative bacteria whereas others are tested with both?

SECTION 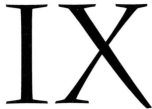 Microbiology of the
Intestinal Tract

EXERCISE 24 The *Enterobacteriaceae* (Enteric Bacilli)

Reference: Morello, Mizer, Wilson, and Granato, Microbiology in Patient Care, 5th edition, 1994. Chapter 16.

The human intestinal tract is inhabited from birth by a variety of microorganisms acquired, at first, from the mother. Later, organisms are carried in with food and water or introduced by hands and other objects placed in the mouth. Once inside, many succumb to the acid conditions encountered in the stomach or the activity of digestive enzymes in the upper part of the intestinal tract. The small intestine and lower bowel, however, offer appropriate conditions for survival and multiplication of many microorganisms, primarily *anaerobic* species, that live there without harming their host.

When feces are cultured on bacteriologic media, it becomes apparent that most *facultatively aerobic* bacterial species normally inhabiting the intestinal tract are gram-negative, nonsporing bacilli with some culture characteristics in common. This group of organisms is known as "enteric bacilli," or, in taxonomic terms, the family *Enterobacteriaceae*. However, some of the bacterial species that are classified within this group are important agents of intestinal disease. These usually are acquired through ingestion and are referred to as "enteric pathogens." The anaerobic organisms play little role in enteric disease and are not recovered in routine fecal cultures because they require special techniques for isolation (see Exercise 28).

In the experiments of this exercise we shall first study some of the cultural characteristics of those enteric bacilli that normally inhabit the bowel, and then apply this knowledge to understanding the methods used for isolating and identifying the important enteric pathogens.

The gram-negative enteric bacilli are not fastidious organisms. They grow rapidly and well under aerobic conditions on most nutrient media. The use of selective and differential culture media plays a large role in their isolation and identification. Their response to suppressive agents incorporated in culture media, and their specific use of carbohydrate or protein components in the media, provide the key to sorting and identifying them (review the exercises in Section VII).

EXPERIMENT 24.1 Identification of Pure Cultures of *Enterobacteriaceae* from the Normal Intestinal Flora

Purpose	To learn how enteric bacilli are identified biochemically
Materials	Slants of triple-sugar iron agar (TSI)
	SIM tubes
	MR-VP broths
	Slants of Simmons citrate agar
	Urea broths
	Slants of phenylalanine agar
	Lysine and ornithine decarboxylase broths
	Mineral oil in dropper bottle
	Sterile 1.0-ml pipettes
	Pipette bulb or other aspiration device
	Sterile empty test tubes
	Xylene
	Kovac's reagent
	Methyl red indicator
	5% alphanaphthol
	40% sodium or potassium hydroxide
	10% ferric chloride
	Nutrient agar slant cultures of *Escherichia coli, Citrobacter diversus, Klebsiella pneumoniae,* pigmented and nonpigmented *Serratia marcescens, Enterobacter aerogenes, Proteus vulgaris,* and *Providencia stuartii*

Procedures

1. Each student will be assigned two of the nutrient agar slant cultures. Inoculate each culture into the following media:

   TSI (using a straight wire inoculating needle, stab the butt of the tube and streak the slant; the closure should not be tight)
   SIM tubed agar (stab 1/4 of the depth of the medium)
   MR-VP broth
   Simmons citrate agar slant
   Urea broth
   Phenylalanine agar slant
   Lysine decarboxylase broth
   Ornithine decarboxylase broth

2. Carefully overlay the surfaces of the lysine and ornithine broths with 1/2 inch of mineral oil.
3. Incubate all subcultures at 35°C for 24 hours.
4. Before returning to class, read the following descriptions of the biochemical reactions to be observed and instructions for performing them.

Biochemical Reactions and Principles

A. TSI.   TSI contains glucose, lactose, and sucrose as well as a pH-sensitive color indicator. It also contains an iron ingredient for detecting hydrogen sulfide production, which blackens the medium if it occurs (compare with H_2S detection in SIM medium).

Fermentation of the sugars by the test organism is interpreted by the following color changes in the butt and the slant of the medium.

Butt		Slant		
Color	*Reaction*	*Color*	*Reaction*	*Interpretation*
Yellow	Acid	Yellow	Acid	Glucose and lactose and/or sucrose fermented
Yellow	Acid	Orange-red or pink	Neutral or alkaline	Glucose only fermented
Orange-red	Neutral	Orange-red	Neutral	No fermentation
	Bubbles			Gas production

B. IMViC Reactions.   The term **IMViC** is a mnemonic for four reactions: the letter **I** stands for the *indole test,* **M** for the *methyl red test,* **V** for the *Voges-Proskauer* reaction (with a small *i* added to make a pronounceable word), and **C** for citrate.

The *indole test* for tryptophan utilization was described in Experiment 17.3. Perform it in the same way here, using xylene and Kovac's reagent added to SIM cultures.

Methyl red is an acid-sensitive dye that is yellow at a pH above 4.5 and red at a pH below 4.5. When the dye is added to a culture of organisms growing in glucose broth, its color indicates whether the glucose has been broken down completely to highly acidic end products with a pH below 4.5 (methyl red *positive,* red), or only partially to less acidic end products with a pH above 4.5 (methyl red *negative,* yellow).

The *Voges-Proskauer test* can be performed on the same glucose broth culture used for the methyl red test (MR-VP broth). One of the glucose fermentation end products produced by some organisms is acetylmethylcarbinol. The VP reagents (alphanaphthol and potassium hydroxide solutions) oxidize this compound to diacetyl, which in turn reacts with a substance in the broth to form a new compound having a pink to red color. VP-*positive* organisms are those reacting in the test to give this pink color change.

To perform the MR and VP tests, first withdraw 1.0 ml of the MR-VP broth culture, place this in an empty sterile tube, and set the tube aside for the VP test. Discard the pipette in disinfectant.

Do a methyl red test by adding 5 drops of methyl red indicator to 5.0 ml of MR-VP broth culture. Observe and record the color of the dye.

Perform a VP test by adding 0.6 ml of alphanaphthol and 0.2 ml of KOH solutions to 1.0 ml of MR-VP broth culture. Shake the tube well and allow it to stand for 10 to 20 minutes. Observe and record the color.

Citrate can serve some organisms as a sole source of carbon for their metabolic processes, but others require organic carbon sources. The citrate agar used in this test contains bromthymol blue, a dye indicator that turns from green to deep blue in color when bacterial growth occurs. If no growth occurs, the medium remains green in color and the test is negative.

C. Motility and H₂S Production. These properties are observed in SIM cultures, as described in Experiment 17.3.

D. Urease Production. The test for urease was described in Experiment 18.1. Read and record the results of your cultures tested in urea broth.

E. Phenylalanine Deaminase (PD). The test for production of this enzyme was described in Experiment 18.5. Perform it in the same way, adding ferric chloride solution to your cultures on phenylalanine agar medium.

F. Lysine (LD) and Ornithine (OD) Decarboxylases. Lysine and ornithine are amino acids that can be broken down by decarboxylase enzymes possessed by some bacteria. During this process, the carboxyl (COOH) group on the amino acid molecule is removed, leaving alkaline end products that change the color of the pH indicator. In the broth test you use, a positive test is a deep purple color; a negative test is yellow. The reactions work best when air is excluded from the medium; therefore, the broths are layered with mineral oil after inoculation and before incubation.

Results

Record results for your cultures in the following table. Obtain results for other cultures by observing those assigned to fellow students.

Genus of Organism	TSI		I	M	Vi	C	H₂S	Motility	Urease[†]	PD	LD	OD
	Slant*	Butt*										
Escherichia												
Citrobacter												
Klebsiella												
Enterobacter												
Serratia[‡] 1												
Serratia[‡] 2												
Proteus												
Providencia												

*A = acid; K = neutral or alkaline; G = gas.

[†]If positive, specify time.

[‡]1 = pigmented strain; 2 = nonpigmented strain.

EXPERIMENT 24.2   Isolation Techniques for Enteric Pathogens

Bacterial diseases of the intestinal tract can be highly communicable and may spread in epidemic fashion. Their agents enter the body through the mouth in contaminated food or water, or as a result of direct contacts with infected persons. Among the *Enterobacteriaceae,* the organisms of pathogenic significance belong to the genera *Salmonella, Shigella,* and *Yersinia.* Also certain *Escherichia coli* strains can produce disease by several mechanisms including invading tissue or producing toxins. Such strains are referred to as enteroinvasive or enterotoxigenic, respectively.

The many species of *Salmonella* can be distinguished on the basis of their serological properties as well as their biochemical activities. These organisms characteristically cause acute gastroenteritis when ingested, but some also can find their way into other body tissues and cause systemic disease. Among these, the most important is *Salmonella typhi,* the agent of typhoid fever, a serious systemic infection. The salmonellae are gram-negative bacilli that are usually motile. They usually do not ferment lactose but display a variety of other fermentative and enzymatic activities.

Shigella species are the agents of bacillary dysentery. These organisms are gram-negative and nonmotile. They usually do not ferment lactose. In fermenting other carbohydrates they produce acid but not gas (with one exception). They can also be identified to species by serological methods.

Yersinia enterocolitica is the cause of acute enterocolitis, primarily in children. Its symptoms may mimic those produced by *Salmonella, Shigella,* or enteroinvasive *E. coli.* Occasionally, the symptoms are more suggestive of acute appendicitis. The organism grows better at room temperature (25°C) than at 35°C; therefore, it may not be isolated unless the physician notifies the laboratory that yersiniosis is suspected. In this case the isolation plates are incubated at both temperatures. *Yersinia* are gram-negative bacilli that are motile at 25°C but not at 35°C. They ferment sucrose, but not lactose. *Y. enterocolitica* is urease positive.

Disease-producing *E. coli* were once thought to be associated only with epidemic diarrhea in babies, but they are now known to be a common cause of "traveler's diarrhea" ("turista") and a variety of other gastrointestinal diseases. Some of these strains may be distinguished from others by immunological typing.

The pathogenic *Enterobacteriaceae* are first isolated from clinical specimens by using highly selective media to suppress the normal flora in feces and to allow the pathogens to grow. Many of these media contain lactose, with a pH indicator, to differentiate the lactose-nonfermenting *Salmonella, Shigella,* and *Yersinia* (colorless on these agars) from any lactose-fermenting normal flora that may survive (pink or red colonies, see colorplate 16). EMB or MacConkey agar is commonly used, together with two more highly selective media such as Hektoen enteric (HE) and bismuth sulfite (BiS) agars. In addition, an "enrichment" broth containing suppressants for normal enteric flora is inoculated. After an incubation period to allow enteric pathogens to multiply, the enrichment broth is subcultured onto selective and differential agar plates to permit isolation of the pathogen from among the suppressed normal flora. Subsequent identification procedures are based on the same types of biochemical tests that you have studied, but may be more extensive to differentiate the enzymatic activities of enteric species that are closely related to *Salmonella* or *Shigella.*

Other bacterial pathogens are associated with intestinal disease. *Campylobacter jejuni,* a curved, gram-negative bacillus, may be the most common bacterial agent of diarrhea in children and young adults (see colorplate 6). It has relatively strict growth requirements and special procedures must be used to isolate it in the laboratory. Some vibrios, notably *Vibrio cholerae* (the agent of cholera) and *Vibrio parahaemolyticus* (of the family *Vibrionaceae*), represent other examples of significant intestinal tract pathogens. These organisms can also be isolated from cultures of fecal material and identified by their characteristic morphological and metabolic properties. Although the choice of isolation media and identification procedures must be varied according to the nature of the organism being sought in a specimen, the principles are the same as those we are following here. You should read further about infectious diseases acquired through the intestinal tract, including bacterial food poisonings, and be prepared to discuss the essential features of their laboratory diagnosis, beginning with the collection of appropriate specimens.

Figure 24.1 Flowchart showing procedures for isolation and initial identification of *Enterobacteriaceae*.

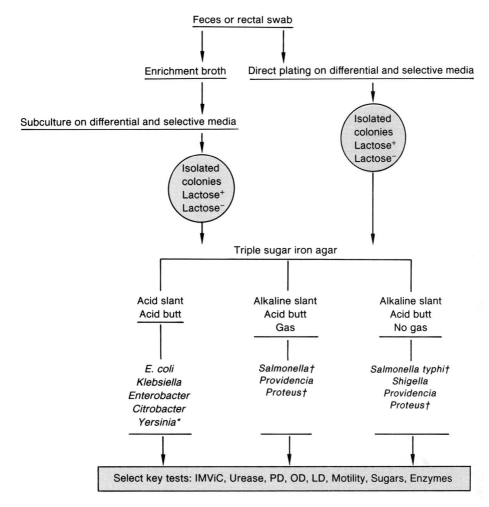

Feces or rectal swab

Enrichment broth

Direct plating on differential and selective media

Subculture on differential and selective media

Isolated colonies Lactose⁺ Lactose⁻

Isolated colonies Lactose⁺ Lactose⁻

Triple sugar iron agar

Acid slant
Acid butt

E. coli
Klebsiella
Enterobacter
Citrobacter
Yersinia*

Alkaline slant
Acid butt
Gas

Salmonella†
Providencia
Proteus†

Alkaline slant
Acid butt
No gas

Salmonella typhi†
Shigella
Providencia
Proteus†

Select key tests: IMViC, Urease, PD, OD, LD, Motility, Sugars, Enzymes

*Although *Yersinia* is lactose negative, it is sucrose positive.
†H₂S produced

In this experiment, and the one that follows, we shall review the basic methods for isolation and identification of enteric pathogens belonging to the genera *Salmonella* and *Shigella*. The general procedures are summarized in the flowchart shown in figure 24.1, and the biochemical reactions that you have studied in identifying *Enterobacteriaceae* are reviewed in table 24.3-1.

Purpose	To observe the morphology of *Salmonella* and *Shigella* species on selective and differential isolation plates
Materials	EMB or MacConkey plates Hektoen enteric (HE) plates Bismuth sulfite (BiS) agar plates Agar slant cultures of a *Salmonella* species and a *Shigella* species

Table 24.3-1 *Enterobacteriaceae*

Important Genera	Pathogenicity	Lactose	I	M	Vi	C	Motility	H₂S	Urea	PD	LD	OD
Salmonella	Typhoid fever Gastroenteritis	−	−	+	−	+	+	+	−	−	+	+†
Shigella	Bacillary dysentery	− or late	±*	+	−	−	−	−	−	−	−	±
Escherichia	Normal flora in GI tract Urinary tract infection Infant and traveler's diarrhea	+	+	+	−	−	±	−	−	−	+	±
Citrobacter	Normal flora Urinary tract infection	+	−	+	−	+	±	±	−	−	−	±
Klebsiella	Respiratory infection Urinary tract infection	+	−	−	+	+	−	−	+ late	−	+	−
Enterobacter	Normal flora Urinary tract infection	+	−	−	+	+	+	−	− or late	−	+	+
Serratia	Normal flora Urinary tract infection Nosocomial infection	− or late	−	−	+	+	+	−	−	−	+	+
Proteus	Normal flora Urinary tract infection	−	±	+	±	±	+	±	+ rapid	+	−	±
Providencia	Normal flora Urinary tract infection	−	+	+	−	+	+	−	−	+	−	−
Yersinia	Gastroenteritis Mesenteric adenitis	−	±	+	−	−	+ (25°C) −(35°C)	−	+	−	−	+

*± = Some species or strains +, some −

†*S. typhi* is OD negative

Procedures

1. Inoculate a *Salmonella* culture on each of the selective media provided. Streak for isolation. Do the same with a *Shigella* culture.
2. Incubate your six plates at 35°C for 24 hours. Continue the incubation of BiS plates for 48 hours.
3. Examine all plates and record your observations under Results.

Results

Name of Organism	Colonial Morphology on			
	EMB	MacConkey	HE	BiS
Salmonella				
Shigella				

Look up the composition of HE agar. List the major ingredients and state why you think they should affect the appearance of *Salmonella* in the way you have reported.

EXPERIMENT **24.3**   **Identification Techniques for Enteric Pathogens**

Purpose	To study some biochemical reactions of *Salmonella* and *Shigella*
Materials	TSI slants
	SIM tubes
	MR-VP broths
	Simmons citrate slants
	Urea broth tubes
	Phenylalanine agar slants
	Lysine and ornithine decarboxylase broths
	Mineral oil in dropper bottle
	Sterile 1.0-ml pipettes
	Pipette bulb or other aspiration device
	Sterile empty tubes
	Xylene
	Kovac's reagent
	Methyl red indicator
	5% alphanaphthol
	40% sodium or potassium hydroxide
	10% ferric chloride
	Agar slant cultures of *Salmonella* and *Shigella* species

Procedures

1. You will be assigned a culture of either *Salmonella* or *Shigella*. Inoculate one tube of each medium provided, i.e.: TSI; SIM; MR-VP broth; citrate slant; urea, lysine, and ornithine broths; and phenylalanine agar.
2. Incubate all tubes at 35°C for 24 hours.
3. Complete the IMViC and PD tests (see Exp. 24.1). Read and record all biochemical reactions under Results. Observe your neighbors' results and record all information for both organisms.

Results

Name of Organism	TSI		*I*	*M*	*Vi*	*C*	*H₂S*	Motility	Urease	PD	LD	OD
	Slant	Butt										
Salmonella												
Shigella												

EXPERIMENT 24.4 Techniques to Distinguish Nonfermentative Gram-Negative Bacilli from *Enterobacteriaceae*

A variety of gram-negative bacilli that normally inhabit soil and water or live as commensals on human mucous membranes may contaminate specimens sent to the microbiology laboratory for culture or, more importantly, may produce opportunistic human infections. Although the Gram-stain appearance and cultural characteristics of the organisms may resemble those of *Enterobacteriaceae*, they are relatively inactive in the common biochemical tests. In particular, they either fail to metabolize glucose or they degrade it by oxidative rather than fermentative pathways. For this reason these organisms are often referred to as "glucose nonfermenters" (as opposed to the glucose-fermenting enteric bacilli). A number of bacterial genera and species are included in this group of nonfermenters. The most important from a medical aspect is *Pseudomonas aeruginosa*, which is most often involved in human infection. Because of the different clinical implications and the varying antimicrobial susceptibility patterns (nonfermenters are more highly resistant to common antimicrobial agents) it is important to distinguish nonfermenters from enteric bacilli. The characteristics of a few nonfermenting bacteria are listed in table 24.4-1 and compared with those of the *Enterobacteriaceae*.

Table 24.4-1 Characteristics of Nonfermenting Gram-Negative Bacilli

	Butt of TSI	O-F glucose*		Oxidase	Complete Hemolysis	Diffusible Green Pigment
		Open	Closed			
Pseudomonas aeruginosa	No change	+	−	+	+	+
Acinetobacter anitratus	No change	+	−	−	−	−
Acinetobacter lwoffi	No change	−	−	−	−	−
Alcaligenes faecalis	No change	−	−	+	−	−
Enterobacteriaceae	Yellow	+	+	−	− or +	−

*A positive test is a yellow color. Yellow in the open tube only indicates glucose degradation or *oxidation*. A yellow color in the closed tube (with mineral oil) indicates the organism is *fermentative* rather than oxidative. Glucose fermenters produce acid (yellow color) in the open as well as the closed tube.

Purpose	To study some biochemical reactions of glucose nonfermenting bacteria
Materials	Blood agar plates
	Nutrient agar plates
	TSI slant
	O-F glucose deeps
	Oxidase reagent (di- or tetramethyl-*p*-phenylenediamine)
	Dropper bottle with sterile mineral oil
	Slant cultures of *Pseudomonas aeruginosa, Acinetobacter anitratus,* and *Escherichia coli*

Procedures

1. Prepare and examine a Gram stained smear of each organism.
2. Inoculate a blood and nutrient agar plate with each organism. Streak the plate to obtain isolated colonies.
3. Inoculate each organism onto a TSI slant by stabbing the butt and streaking the slant.
4. Inoculate *two* tubes of O-F glucose with each organism by stabbing your inoculating loop to the bottom of the column of medium. Overlay *one* of each set of two tubes with a one-half inch layer of sterile mineral oil.
5. Label all plates and tubes. Incubate them at 35°C for 24 hours.
6. Test each organism for the presence of the enzyme *oxidase*. The procedure is as follows:
   a. Take a sterile petri dish containing a piece of filter paper.
   b. Wet the paper with oxidase reagent.
   c. With your inoculating loop, scrape up some growth from the tube labeled *P. aeruginosa* and rub it on a small area of the wet filter paper. You should see an immediate *positive* oxidase reaction as the color of the area changes from light pink to black-purple.
   d. Repeat procedure 6c using growth from the tubes labeled *A. anitratus* and *E. coli*. Record the results in the table that follows.

Results

1. Examine the blood agar plate for hemolysis and the nutrient agar for pigment production.
2. Read and record all biochemical reactions in the following table:

| Name of Organism | Gram-Stain Appearance | | Butt of TSI | O-F Glucose | | Oxidase | Complete Hemolysis | Diffusible Green Pigment |
	Blood Agar	Nutrient Agar		Open	Closed			
P. aeruginosa								
A. anitratus								
E. coli								

EXPERIMENT 24.5   Rapid Methods for Bacterial Identification

The biochemical tests performed in the preceding sections are representative of standard methods for bacterial identification. In some instances, it is possible to identify a bacterium correctly by using only a few tests, but more often an extensive biochemical "profile" is needed. Because it is expensive and time-consuming to make and keep a wide variety of culture media on hand, many microbiology laboratories now use multimedia identification kits. These are commercially available and are especially useful for identifying the common enteric bacteria. The use of such kits is customarily referred to as an application of "rapid methods," even though they must be incubated overnight, as usual, before results can be read. Some of them, indeed, are rapid to inoculate, while others permit complete identification within 24 hours.

One type of kit, the Enterotube II (Roche Diagnostics, see Appendix III[C]), is a tube of 12 compartmentalized, conventional agar media that can be inoculated rapidly from a single isolated colony on an agar plate (see colorplate 23). The media provided indicate whether the organism ferments the carbohydrates glucose, lactose, adonitol, arabinose, sorbitol, and dulcitol; produces H_2S and/or indole; produces acetylmethylcarbinol; deaminates phenylalanine; splits urea; decarboxylates lysine and/or ornithine; and can use citrate when it is the sole source of carbon in the medium. The mechanism of the other tests provided by the Enterotube II has been described in previous exercises or experiments (17, 18, 24.1).

The API System (Analytab Products, see Appendix III[C]) represents another type of kit for rapid identification of bacteria. This system provides, in a single strip, a series of 20 microtubules (miniature test tubes) of dehydrated media that are rehydrated with a saline suspension of the bacterium to be identified (see colorplate 23). The tests included in the strip determine whether the organism ferments glucose, mannitol, inositol, sorbitol, rhamnose, saccharose, melibiose, and amygdalin; produces indole and H_2S; splits urea; breaks down the amino acids tryptophan (same mechanism as phenylalanine), lysine, ornithine, and arginine; produces gelatinase; forms acetylmethylcarbinol from glucose (VP test); and splits the compound o-nitrophenyl-β-D-galactopyranoside (ONPG). The enzyme that acts on ONPG, called β-galactosidase, also is responsible for lactose fermentation. Some bacteria, however, are unable to transport lactose into their cells for breakdown, although they possess β-galactosidase. In lactose broth, therefore, such bacteria fail to display acid production, or do so only after a delay of days or weeks. By contrast, in ONPG medium their β-galactosidase splits the substrate in a matter of hours, producing a bright yellow end product. Thus, ONPG can be used for the rapid demonstration of an organism's ability to ferment lactose.

A third type of kit is known as the Minitek System (Becton Dickinson Microbiology Systems, see Appendix III[C]). This is a miniaturized differentiation system that consists of filter paper disks (similar to antimicrobial disks) impregnated with biochemical substrates, and a plastic plate containing 12 wells. A different disk is dispensed into each well. Each disk is then hydrated with a measured amount of a broth suspension of the organism to be identified. About 35 different substrates (to detect sugar fermentations, amino acid decarboxylations, H_2S production, and so on) are available on Minitek disks. This system differs from the other two in that the microbiologist can choose only those tests desired by selecting appropriate disks for placement in the wells of the plastic dish.

In order to permit more accurate bacterial identification, a computerized recognition system has been devised for each of these three kits that assigns a number to each positive biochemical reaction. These figures are grouped together to give a numerical code to each organism. Unknown bacteria can be identified by looking up the code number provided by their positive reactions in an index book. Different strains of the same bacterium may vary in certain biochemical test results and thus have different code numbers. These variations can sometimes be used as epidemiological markers, in much the same way as phage typing is used to recognize different strains of *Staphylococcus aureus.*

A further advance is the use of *automated* instruments to read and interpret the results of both identification and antimicrobial susceptibility tests. The tests are set up in special, clear plastic multiwelled chambers containing a battery of biochemicals and different concentrations of several antimicrobial agents. The plastic chambers are then incubated in the instrument, which periodically scans each biochemical well for changes in the color of pH indicators and scans the antimicrobial agent wells for the presence of turbidity (signifying resistance). At the end of a specific time period, the computer in the instrument interprets all reactions and then the organism identification and its antimicrobial susceptibility results are printed out. Depending on the system used, results can be obtained in as little as two to six hours.

In this experiment some rapid nonautomated methods for identification of bacteria will be demonstrated.

Purpose	To observe the biochemical properties of bacteria grown in a multimedia system for rapid identification
Materials	Two Enterotubes, API strips, or Minitek plates (as available) inoculated, respectively, with *Escherichia coli* and *Proteus vulgaris,* and incubated for 24 hours. The instructor will demonstrate methods for completing each test in the system.

Results

1. If Enterotubes were inoculated, record the results observed for each organism in the blocks provided under the following diagram:

	Dextrose	Lysine	Ornithine	H₂S/ indole	Adon-itol	Lactose	Arabi-nose	Sorbitol	Voges-Proskauer	Dulcitol PAD	Urea	Citrate
Uninoculated colors	Red / orange	Yellow	Yellow	Yellow	Red / orange	Red / orange	Red / orange	Red / orange	Colorless	Green	Yellow	Green
Reacted colors	Yellow	Purple	Purple	H₂S-black Indole--red†	Yellow	Yellow	Yellow	Yellow	Red†	Dulcitol--yellow PAD--brown	Pink	Blue
E. coli (+ or −)				H₂S: Ind.:						Dulc: PAD:		
P. vulgaris (+ or −)				H₂S: Ind.:						Dulc: PAD:		

Roche Diagnostic Systems.

*If this wax overlay is separated from the dextrose agar surface, gas has been produced by the organism.
†Requires addition of indole or Voges-Proskauer reagents.

2. If API strips were inoculated, record the results observed for each organism in the blocks provided under the following diagram:

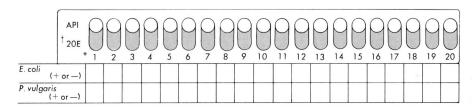

API †20E *	1	2	3	4	5	6	7	8	9	10	11	12	13	14	15	16	17	18	19	20
E. coli (+ or −)																				
P. vulgaris (+ or −)																				

*Code	Test	Negative Reaction	Positive Reaction
1—ONPG	ONPG	Colorless	Yellow
2—ADH	Arginine dihydrolase	Yellow	Red or orange
3—LDC	Lysine decarboxylase	Yellow	Red or orange
4—ODC	Ornithine decarboxylase	Yellow	Red or orange
5—CIT	Citrate	Light green or yellow	Blue
6—H₂S	Hydrogen sulfide	No black deposit	Black deposit
7—URE	Urea	Yellow	Red or orange
8—TDA	Tryptophan deaminase	Yellow	Brown-red
9—IND	Indole	Yellow	Red-ring
10—VP	Voges-Proskauer	Colorless	Red within 10 min.
11—GEL	Gelatin	No black pigment diffusion	Black pigment diffusion
12—GLU	Glucose	Blue or blue-green	Yellow or gray
13—MAN	Mannitol	Blue or blue-green	Yellow
14—INO	Inositol	Blue or blue-green	Yellow
15—SOR	Sorbitol	Blue or blue-green	Yellow
16—RHA	Rhamnose	Blue or blue-green	Yellow
17—SAC	Saccharose	Blue or blue-green	Yellow
18—MEL	Melibiose	Blue or blue-green	Yellow
19—AMY	Amygdalin	Blue or blue-green	Yellow
20—ARA	Arabinose	Blue or blue-green	Yellow

†20 E = 20-test strip for enteric bacteria.

3. If the Minitek system was used, complete the following table:

Disk Substrate (Test) Used	Negative Reaction	Positive Reaction	E. coli (+ or −)	P. vulgaris (+ or −)
1.				
2.				
3.				
4.				
5.				
6.				
7.				
8.				
9.				
10.				
11.				
12.				

Questions

1. What does the term IMViC mean?

2. Why is the IMViC useful in identifying *Enterobacteriaceae?* Are further biochemical tests necessary for complete identification?

3. What diagnostic test differentiates *Proteus* and *Providencia* species from other *Enterobacteriaceae?*

4. How is *E. coli* distinguished from *P. vulgaris* on MacConkey agar? On a TSI slant?

5. Instead of TSI, why would a slant medium containing only dextrose and lactose (not sucrose) be preferable for detecting *Y. enterocolitica?*

6. What procedures, other than biochemical, are used to identify microorganisms?

7. Describe two mechanisms by which *E. coli* can produce disease.

8. What is meant by the term "enteric pathogen"?

9. Name a bacterial pathogen, other than one of the *Enterobacteriaceae,* that causes intestinal disease. Provide a flowchart indicating how you would make the laboratory diagnosis.

10. Name a rapid method for the identification of *Enterobacteriaceae,* and discuss its value in comparison with the methods you have used in Exercise 24.

11. Why is it important to differentiate glucose nonfermenters from *Enterobacteriaceae?*

EXERCISE 25 Clinical Specimens from the Intestinal Tract

Reference: Morello, Mizer, Wilson, and Granato, Microbiology in Patient Care, 5th edition, 1994.
Chapter 16.

This exercise provides you with an opportunity to apply your knowledge of the *Enterobacteriaceae* to making a laboratory diagnosis of an intestinal infection. In the first experiment you will prepare a culture of your own feces and observe the normal intestinal flora on primary isolation plates. In the second experiment you will be given a pure culture of one of the *Enterobacteriaceae* as an "unknown" to be identified. The third experiment is an antimicrobial susceptibility test of your pure unknown culture. Here you should observe the differences in response of gram-negative enteric bacilli, as compared with streptococci and staphylococci studied earlier, to the most clinically useful antimicrobial agents.

EXPERIMENT 25.1 Culturing a Fecal Sample

Purpose	To study some enteric bacilli normally found in the bowel
Materials	A stool specimen
	Swab
	Tubed sterile saline (0.5 ml)
	EMB or MacConkey agar plate
	Hektoen enteric (HE) agar plate
	Blood agar plate

Procedures

1. Bring a *fresh* sample of your feces to the laboratory session. Collect it in a clean container fitted with a tight lid (a screw-cap jar; waxed, cardboard cup; or plastic vessel).
2. Using a swab, take up about 1 gm of feces (a piece the size of a large pea) and emulsify this in the tube of saline.
3. Inoculate the fecal suspension, with the swab, on a blood agar, EMB or MacConkey agar plate, and a Hektoen enteric (HE) plate. Discard the swab in disinfectant solution. Streak for isolation, using a loop.
4. Incubate the plates at 35°C for 24 hours.

Results

1. Describe the appearance of growth on your plate cultures:

Plate	Relative Number of Colonies	Number of Colony Types	Color of Colonies	Hemolysis
Blood agar				
EMB or MacConkey				X
HE				X

2. Interpret any difference in numbers of colonies on these plates.

3. Interpret the color of colonies on EMB or MacConkey agar.

4. Interpret the appearance of colonies on the HE plate.

5. Were any lactose-negative colonies present? If so, name the genera to which they might belong and indicate the key procedures that would identify each.

EXPERIMENT **25.2**   **Identification of an Unknown Enteric Organism**

| **Purpose** | To use the techniques you have learned to identify an unknown pure culture |
| **Materials** | Same as in Experiments 24.2 and 24.3 except that your assigned culture is numbered, not labeled |

Procedures

1. Prepare a Gram stain of your culture.
2. Inoculate the culture on EMB or MacConkey, HE, and BiS plates, and streak for isolation.
3. Inoculate all tubed media provided.
4. Incubate plates and tubes at 35°C for 24 hours.

Results

Read and record your results across one line of the following table. Also record all results obtained by your neighbors with different strains. Using table 24.3-1, identify the unknown organisms.

Specimen Number	Gram-Stain Reaction and Morphology	EMB	MacConkey	Bismuth Sulfite	HE	TSI	I	M	Vi	C	H₂S	Motility	Urea	PD	LD	OD	Identification

Clinical Specimens from the Intestinal Tract

EXPERIMENT 25.3   Antimicrobial Susceptibility Test of an Enteric Organism

Purpose	To determine the antimicrobial susceptibility pattern of a gram-negative enteric bacillus
Materials	Nutrient agar plates (Mueller-Hinton if available)
	Antimicrobial disks
	Sterile swabs
	Forceps
	Beaker containing 70% alcohol
	Pure plate or slant culture of unknown from Experiment 25.2
	Tube of nutrient broth (5.0 ml)

Procedures

1. Using a sterile swab or inoculating loop, take some of the growth of the pure culture of your unknown organism and emulsify it in 5.0 ml of nutrient broth to equal the turbidity of a McFarland 0.5 standard. (Discard the swab.)
2. Take another sterile swab, dip it in the broth suspension, drain off excess fluid against the inner wall of the tube.
3. Inoculate an agar plate as described in Experiment 15.1.
4. Follow procedures 4 through 7 of Experiment 15.1.
5. Incubate the agar plate at 35°C for 24 hours.
6. Examine plates and record results for each antimicrobial disk as S (susceptible), MS (moderately susceptible), I (intermediate), or R (resistant).
7. Compare results with those obtained for the organism you tested in Experiment 15.1 and Experiment 23.3.

Results

Record your findings:

Antimicrobial Agent	Organism in Exp. 15.1 Name:	S	MS	I	R	Organism in Exp. 23.3 Name:	S	MS	I	R	Organism in Exp. 25.3 Name:	S	MS	I	R

1. Judging by the results of your tests, what group of antimicrobial agents appear to be indicated for the treatment of patients with gram-negative infections? Gram-positive infections?

2. What conclusions can you draw as to the importance of testing each suspected bacterial pathogen for its antimicrobial susceptibility?

Questions

1. What diseases are caused by *Salmonella?*

2. How do salmonellae enter the body? From what sources?

3. Name two selective media for the isolation of *Salmonella* and *Shigella.*

4. Name some of the normal flora of the intestinal tract.

5. Why is it not necessary to collect a stool for culture in a sterile container?

6. How did you dispose of the fecal specimen after inoculating cultures? How should the cultures be disposed of? Why?

7. Were the organisms in your fecal culture predominantly lactose fermenters or nonfermenters? Does this have significance?

8. How do intestinal flora gain entry to the body?

9. Are the gram-negative enteric bacilli fastidious organisms? Would they survive well outside of the body? If so, what significance would this have in their transmission?

SECTION 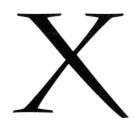 Microbiology of the
Urinary and Genital Tracts

EXERCISE 26   Urine Culture Techniques

Reference: Morello, Mizer, Wilson, and Granato, Microbiology in Patient Care, *5th edition, 1994.*
Chapters 4, 21.

Normally, urine is sterile when excreted by the kidneys and stored in the urinary bladder. When it is voided, however, urine becomes contaminated by the normal flora of the urethra and other superficial urogenital membranes. The presence of bacteria in voided urine (*bacteriuria*), therefore, does not always indicate urinary tract infection. To confirm infection, either the numbers of organisms present or the species isolated must be shown to be significant.

Active infection of the urinary tract arises in one of three ways: (1) microorganisms circulating in the bloodstream from another site of infection are deposited and multiply in the kidneys to produce *pyelonephritis* by the *hematogenous* (originating from the blood) *route;* (2) bacteria colonizing the external urogenital surfaces ascend the urethra to the bladder, causing *cystitis* (infection of the bladder only) or pyelonephritis by the *ascending route;* or (3) microorganisms, usually from the urethra, find their way into the bladder on catheters or cystoscopes.

Cystitis is much more common than pyelonephritis. In the former case, most of the offending organisms are opportunistic members of the fecal flora, including many you have studied in the previous two exercises, e.g., *E. coli* (by far the most frequent cause of urinary tract infection), *Klebsiella, Enterobacter, Serratia,* and *Proteus. Pseudomonas* and enterococci are also often incriminated, especially in hospitalized patients with indwelling urinary catheters or those receiving multiple antimicrobial agents. When these nonfastidious organisms reach the bladder, where active host defense mechanisms (blood phagocytes and antibodies) are not readily available, they may grow in the urine, producing acute bladder and urethral symptoms (urgency; frequent, painful urination).

The blood that flows through the kidneys normally carries no microorganisms because phagocytic white blood cells and serum antibodies are constantly at work eliminating any microbial intruders that reach deep tissues. If these defense mechanisms are not working well or become overwhelmed by extensive infectious processes in systemic tissues (uncontrolled tuberculosis or yeast infections, staphylococcal or streptococcal abscesses), then the kidneys may become infected by organisms carried to them via the bloodstream. More commonly, however, microorganisms initially colonizing the bladder ascend the ureters to infect the kidneys.

Laboratory diagnosis of urinary tract infections is made by culturing urine, usually obtained either by catheterization or by voided collection. Catheterized urine is not contaminated by normal urogenital flora, but the technique itself may introduce organisms into the bladder. For this reason, catheters are seldom used to collect routinely ordered urine cultures. In culturing voided specimens, however, the laboratory is faced with several problems. One is the normal contamination of voided urine; another is the need for speed in initiating culture before contaminants can multiply and distort results; and a third is the obligation to obtain and report results that reflect the clinical problem adequately and accurately. Contamination by hardy, nonfastidious organisms can mask the presence of other pathogens that are difficult to cultivate on artificial media. Overgrowths in standing urine give a false picture of numbers. Either situation can lead to laboratory results that fail to reveal the clinical problem, and possibly to the mismanagement of the patient's case.

To meet these problems, the laboratory must insist on proper techniques for urine collection and on prompt delivery of specimens for culture. When delay is unavoidable, urine specimens should be refrigerated to prevent multiplication of any microorganisms they may contain. Upon receipt in the laboratory, the urine is examined for certain physical properties that can indicate infection, e.g., color, odor, turbidity, pH, mucus, blood, or pus. Uncontaminated urine is usually clear, but sometimes may be clouded with precipitating salts. Urine containing actively multiplying bacteria is turbid. If the patient has a urinary tract infection, the urine usually also contains many white blood cells. A direct Gram stain may be useful in providing an estimate of the kinds and numbers of bacteria or cells present. In some instances, the mere finding of a pathogenic bacterial species in urine (e.g., *Salmonella, Mycobacterium tuberculosis,* or beta-hemolytic streptococci) is significant, regardless of numbers, and the search for such organisms does not require quantitative culture technique. It is generally advisable, however, to culture urine quantitatively, and to report a "colony count"—that is, the numbers of colonies that grow in culture from a measured quantity of urine. If microorganisms are actively colonizing the kidneys or bladder, they can usually be demonstrated in large numbers in urine (in excess of

100,000 organisms per milliliter of urine). On the other hand, normal urine that is merely contaminated in passage down the urethra contains very few organisms (100 to 1,000 per milliliter, not more than 10,000), *provided* it is cultured soon after collection, before multiplication of contaminants can occur in the voided specimen awaiting culture. Some patients with symptoms of cystitis have low counts of the causative agent in their urine and close collaboration between the laboratory and the physician is needed to accurately diagnose these infections.

Collection of voided urine for culture ("clean-catch" techniques)

Aseptic urine collection requires careful cleansing of the external urogenital surfaces, using gauze sponges moistened with tap water and liquid soap.

For males, the procedure simply entails thorough sponging of the penis, discard of the first stream of urine, and collection of a "midstream" portion in a sterile container fitted with a leak-proof closure. If the outside of the container has been soiled in the process, it must be wiped clean with disinfectant before being handled further.

For females, extra care is necessary. All labial surfaces must be thoroughly cleansed, and the sterile container must be held in such a way that it does not come in contact with the skin or clothing. Again, the first stream of urine is discarded, and a midstream sample is collected. When the container has been tightly closed, it is wiped clean with disinfectant.

Urine containers should never be filled to the brim. Closures should be double-checked to make certain they will not permit leakage during transport to the laboratory. If there is any delay (*before* or *after* delivery to the lab) in initiating culture, *urine specimens must be refrigerated.*

EXPERIMENT **26.1** **Examination and Qualitative Culture of Voided Urine**

Purpose	To learn simple urine culture technique and to appreciate the value of aseptic urine collection
Materials	Sterile urine collection vessels
	Liquid soap
	Sterile gauze sponges
	Sterile empty test tubes
	Sterile 5.0-ml pipettes
	Pipette bulb or other aspiration device
	Litmus or pH papers
	Blood agar plates
	EMB or MacConkey plates
	Two samples of your own urine

Procedures

1. Without special preparation of the urogenital surfaces, collect a specimen of your urine in a sterile container. Wipe the outside of the container with disinfectant and close it tightly.
2. *Aseptically* collect a second sample of your urine, following appropriate "clean-catch" techniques described in this exercise.
3. If possible, these specimens should be collected *within one hour* of the start of the laboratory session. If they are collected earlier, *refrigerate them.*
4. Place about 1.0 ml of each urine sample in a small sterile test tube. Hold the tubes to the light and examine urine for color and turbidity. Test the pH of each sample with litmus or pH paper. Note the odor of each. Record your observations under Results.
5. Going back to the original urine container (the test tube sample is now contaminated by the pH test), pipette a large drop of the "clean-catch" specimen onto a blood agar plate near the edge, and another drop onto an EMB or MacConkey plate. Spread the drop a little with your loop and then streak for isolation.

6. Repeat procedure 5 with the casual urine collection.
7. Incubate all plates at 35°C for 24 hours.
8. Examine the incubated plates for amount of growth, types of colonies, and microscopic morphology of colony types. Record observations under Results.

Results

1. Macroscopic appearance of urine:

Specimen	Color	Turbidity	Odor	Clots	pH
Clean catch					
Casual					

2. Culture results:

Specimen	Blood Agar			EMB or MacConkey		
	Amount of Growth	Types of Colonies	Gram Morphology	Amount of Growth	Types of Colonies	Gram Morphology
Clean catch						
Casual						

Interpret any differences you observed in the *amount* of growth recovered from the two specimens.

Interpret differences in the *amount* of growth on blood agar and MacConkey plates for each specimen.

Interpret differences in the *nature* of growth obtained on blood agar and MacConkey plates for each specimen.

Interpret any finding of "no growth."

To distinguish contamination of urine by normal urogenital flora from urinary tract infection by the same organisms, it is usually necessary to determine the numbers of organisms present per milliliter of specimen. In general, counts in excess of *100,000 organisms per milliliter* are considered to indicate *significant bacteriuria,* if the collection technique was adequate and there was no delay in culturing the specimen.

A quantitative culture is prepared by placing a measured volume of urine on an agar plate and counting the number of colonies that develop after incubation. A standardized loop that delivers 0.01 ml of sample is used to inoculate the plate. The number of colonies that appear from this 1/100th-ml sample is multiplied by 100 to give the number per milliliter. For example, if 15 colonies are obtained from 0.01 ml, there are 15 $\times$ 100, or 1,500, organisms present in 1 ml (assuming each colony represents one organism).

In this experiment, you will have a simulated urine specimen from a suspected case of urinary tract infection submitted with a request for quantitative culture.

Purpose	To learn quantitative culture technique and to see the effects of delay in culturing a voided urine specimen
Materials	Nutrient agar plates Standardized loop (0.01-ml delivery) Sterile 5-ml pipettes Pipette bulb or other aspiration device Sterile empty tubes Simulated "clean-catch" urine from a clinical case of urinary tract infection

Procedures

1. With the standardized loop, transfer 0.01 ml of the urine specimen to the center of a nutrient agar plate and streak across the drop in several planes so that the specimen is distributed evenly across the plate.
2. Incubate the plate at 35°C for 24 hours.
3. Go back to the original urine specimen and measure about 2.0 ml into each of two sterile, empty test tubes. Place one of these in the refrigerator, leave one at room temperature at your station, and place the original specimen in the incubator, for 24 hours.
4. Read your plates, count the colonies on each, and report the numbers of organisms per milliliter present in the urine specimen.
5. Inspect the tubes of urine left in the refrigerator, in the incubator, and on your bench. Read for turbidity and record results.

Results

1. Record the number of colonies on the streaked nutrient agar plate.

2. Calculate below the number of organisms per milliliter of specimen and indicate whether this result is significant of urinary tract infection.

3. Diagram your observations of turbidity in each tube of stored urine.

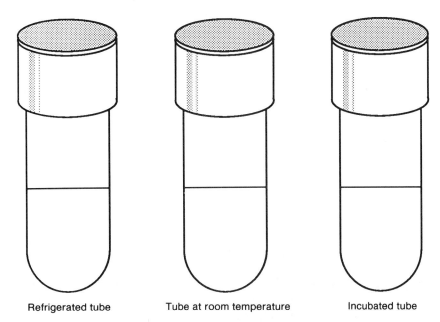

| Refrigerated tube | Tube at room temperature | Incubated tube |

What is your interpretation of the appearance of these tubes?

Questions

1. What is bacteriuria? When is it significant?

2. How do microorganisms enter the urinary tract?

3. Why is aseptic urine collection important when cultures are ordered?

4. List five bacterial species that might be found in an ascending urinary tract infection.

5. If you counted 20 colonies from a 0.01-ml inoculum of a 1:10 dilution of urine, how many organisms per milliliter of specimen would you report? Is this number significant?

6. Is the urine colony count an appropriate indicator of the need for an antimicrobial susceptibility test of an organism isolated from a urine culture? Why?

7. If you took a urine specimen for culture to the laboratory, but found it temporarily closed, what would you do?

8. How would you instruct a female patient to collect her own urine specimen by the "clean-catch" technique? A male patient?

9. What can you learn from visual inspection of a urine specimen?

EXERCISE 27 *Neisseria* and Spirochetes

Reference: Morello, Mizer, Wilson, and Granato, Microbiology in Patient Care, 5th edition, 1994. Chapter 19.

The sexually transmitted diseases are perhaps the most important infections acquired through the urogenital tract, from the social as well as medical point of view. Three frequent infectious diseases of this type are gonorrhea, syphilis, and chlamydial urethritis. All three are caused by bacteria, but chlamydiae require special laboratory techniques for isolation and are described further in Exercise 30. Gonorrhea is caused by *Neisseria gonorrhoeae;* syphilis by *Treponema pallidum,* a spirochete; and chlamydial infection by *Chlamydia trachomatis.*

The bacterial groups to which these sexually transmitted agents belong contain other pathogenic species associated with nonsexually transmitted disease, i.e., infections acquired through other entry portals. Still other species of *Neisseria* and *Treponema* are nonpathogenic, including some that are frequent members of the normal flora of various superficial body membranes.

EXPERIMENT 27.1 *Neisseria*

The genus *Neisseria* contains two pathogenic species and a number of others that are commonly found in the normal flora of the upper respiratory tract. The two medically important species are *N. gonorrhoeae,* the agent of gonorrhea, and *N. meningitidis,* one of the agents of bacterial meningitis. All *Neisseria* are gram-negative diplococci, indistinguishable from each other in microscopic morphology. The pathogenic species are obligate human parasites and quite fastidious in their growth requirements on artificial media. On primary isolation, they require an increased level of CO_2 during incubation at $35°C$. The nonpathogenic commensals of the upper respiratory tract are not fastidious and grow readily on simple nutrient media. Some of the respiratory flora, e.g., *N. subflava* and *N. flavescens,* have a yellow pigment, but most *Neisseria* produce colorless colonies. All *Neisseria* are oxidase positive (see colorplate 13), which helps to distinguish them from other genera, but not from each other. Biochemically, the *Neisseria* species are most readily identified on the basis of their differing patterns of carbohydrate degradation. The differentiation of a few *Neisseria,* including the two pathogenic species, is shown in table 27.1-1.

Gonorrhea usually begins as an acute, local infection of the genital tract. In the male, the urethra is initially involved and exudes a purulent discharge. When the exudate is smeared on a microscope slide and Gram stained, it is seen to contain many polymorphonuclear cells (phagocytic white blood cells), some of which contain intracellular, gram-negative diplococci (see colorplate 4). In the female, acute infection usually begins in the cervix. Smears of the exudate show the same intracellular diplococci as seen in males, except that there are often many more extraneous organisms present in specimens taken from females (see fig. 27.1). Indeed, the abundant normal flora of the vagina may mask the

Table 27.1-1   Differentiation of some *Neisseria* species

Name of Organism	Pathogenicity	Growth on Enriched Media (in CO_2)	Growth on Simple Nutrients (in Air)	Yellow Pigment	Oxidase	Acid Production from*		
						G	M	S
N. gonorrhoeae	Gonorrhea	+	−	−	+	+	−	−
N. meningitidis	Meningitis	+	−	−	+	+	+	−
N. sicca	Normal flora respiratory tract	+	+	±	+	+	+	+
N. flavescens	Normal flora respiratory tract	+	+	+	+	−	−	−

*G = glucose; M = maltose; S = sucrose

Figure 27.1 Diagram of a microscopic field showing intracellular diplococci within polymorphonuclear cells. In cervical smears, organisms of the normal flora may be numerous, but these are extracellular.

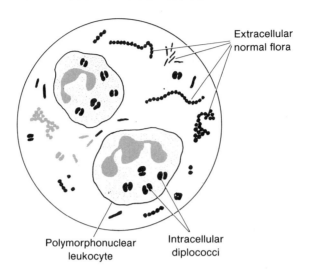

Extracellular
normal flora

Polymorphonuclear
leukocyte

Intracellular
diplococci

presence of gonococci (*N. gonorrhoeae*) in smears or cultures from females. For many women, initial infection may be asymptomatic. Gonococci cannot be demonstrated in smears, and culture techniques *must* be used for laboratory diagnosis. The same situation occurs in a smaller percentage of infected males. Demonstration of *N. gonorrhoeae* in culture provides definitive proof of infection in any case, whether the culture is taken from the cervix, urethra, anus, or throat. When disease is suspected, one or more of these sites should be swabbed for culture, if the patient is a female. If the patient is a male with a urethral discharge, Gram-stained smears of the exudate revealing typical gram-negative intracellular diplococci are considered presumptively diagnostic, and cultures are generally not taken. Figure 27.2 outlines the recommendations of the Centers for Disease Control, U.S. Public Health Service, regarding smears and cultures from males and females, indicating all necessary steps to confirm the diagnosis of gonorrhea.

When cultures are taken, a suitable agar medium should be inoculated directly with the swab, the culture placed in a candle jar or CO_2 incubator and incubated at 35°C pending laboratory examination. Media enriched with hemoglobin and other growth factors are in common use (modified Thayer-Martin and NYC medium are examples). Antimicrobial agents are added to suppress the normal flora of mucous membranes and to make these media more selective for gonococci. Following suitable incubation, laboratory identification of *N. gonorrhoeae* is made by the criteria shown in table 27.1-1.

Meningitis, an inflammation of the meninges of the brain, may be caused by a variety of microbial agents. Chief among them is *Neisseria meningitidis,* a gram-negative diplococcus. The usual portal of entry for these organisms is the upper respiratory tract. They may colonize harmlessly there in the immune individual. When they enter susceptible hosts who cannot keep them localized, they may cause systemic disease, either by finding their way into the bloodstream and then to deep tissues, or by direct extension through the membranous bony structures posterior to the pharynx and sinuses. When they localize on the meninges (the thin membranes that cover the brain), meningococci (*N. meningitidis*) induce an acute, purulent local infection that may have far-reaching effects in the central nervous system. The laboratory diagnosis of *N. meningitidis* infections is made by recovering the organism in cultures of spinal fluid, blood, or the nasopharynx and identifying it by the criteria indicated in table 27.1-1.

In practical situations, it is important to remember that pathogenic *Neisseria* (gonococci and meningococci) are very sensitive to environmental conditions outside the human body, especially temperature and atmosphere. They are easily destroyed in specimens that are (1) delayed in transit to the laboratory, (2) kept at temperatures too far below or above 35°C, (3) heavily contaminated by normal flora, or (4) not promptly provided with an increased CO_2 atmo-

Figure 27.2 Recommended procedures for laboratory diagnosis of gonorrhea. Source: Centers for Disease Control and Prevention, U.S. Public Health Service, Atlanta, Georgia, modified.

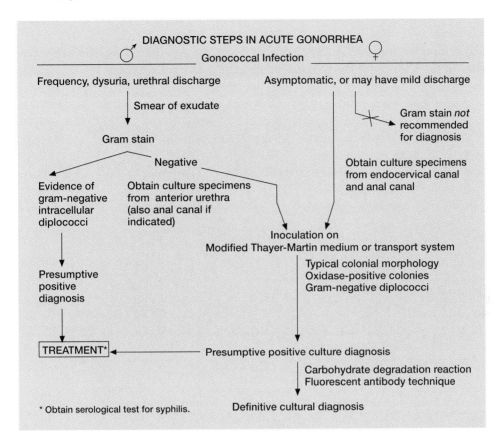

sphere (as in a candle jar). All specimens to be cultured for pathogenic *Neisseria* should be brought *promptly* and *directly* to the microbiologist. If this is not possible, the laboratory's advice should be sought by telephone, while the specimen is still fresh.

In the following experiment, you will have an opportunity to see the cultural and microscopic properties of some *Neisseria* species.

Purpose	To study the microscopic and cultural characteristics of *Neisseria* species

Materials	Sterile petri dish with filter paper
	 Oxidase reagent (dimethyl-*p*-phenylenediamine)
	 Phenol red broths (glucose, maltose, sucrose)
	 Candle jar, containing preincubated chocolate agar plate cultures of:
	    Neisseria sicca (pure culture)
	    Neisseria flavescens (pure culture)
	    A cervical exudate (simulated clinical specimen from a female giving a history of
	       contact with a positive male patient with gonorrhea)
	 Agar slant culture of *E. coli*

Procedures

1. Examine the morphology of colonies on each plate and record their appearance, including pigmentation.
2. Test representative colonies on *each* pure culture plate for the enzyme *oxidase* following the procedure in Experiment 24.4, step 6.
3. Test representative colonies from the plated clinical specimen for their oxidase reactions. Using a wax pencil, mark the bottom of the plate under colonies that are oxidase positive. Record oxidase reactions in the table under Results.
4. Make a Gram stain of an oxidase-positive colony from each of the chocolate plates. Record the microscopic morphology of each in the table under Results.
5. Inoculate one oxidase-positive colony from *each* chocolate agar plate into a glucose, maltose, and sucrose broth tube, respectively.
6. From the plated clinical specimen, select one oxidase-negative colony type (if any) and inoculate it into a glucose, maltose, and sucrose broth tube, respectively.
7. Incubate all carbohydrate subcultures in a candle jar or CO_2 incubator at 35°C for 24 hours. Examine for evidence of acid production. Record results.

Results

1. Record your observations in the table that follows:

Culture	Colonial Morphology	Oxidase (+ or −)	Gram Morphology	Acid production*		
				G	M	S
N. sicca						
N. flavescens						
E. coli				X	X	X
Cervical specimen						
N. gonorrhoeae[†]						
N. meningitidis[†]						

*G = glucose; M = maltose; S = sucrose

[†]To be completed from your reading.

2. Laboratory report of clinical specimen: _____

EXPERIMENT **27.2** **Spirochetes**

The spirochetes are slender, coiled organisms with a longitudinal axial filament that gives them motility. Seen in action, they are long, flexible, and always actively spinning or undulating. Their cell walls are extremely thin and not readily stainable. In unstained wet mounts they are too transparent to be seen by direct condenser light, but become quite visible by "dark-field" condenser illumination. A special condenser lens is used to block the passage of direct light through the mount and to permit only the most oblique rays to enter, at an angle that is nearly parallel to the slide. When viewed in such minimal light, the background of the mount is very dark, almost black, but any particles in suspension are brightly illuminated because they catch and reflect light upward through the objective lens. To stain spirochetes in fixed smears, stains containing metallic precipitates are used. Silver, for example, can be precipitated out of solution and will impregnate spirochetes on the slide, giving them a black color when viewed by ordinary light microscopy (see colorplate 7).

There are three major genera of spirochetes: *Treponema, Borrelia,* and *Leptospira,* each containing species associated with human disease. Many of these organisms are obligate parasites that grow only in human or animal hosts, and others are difficult to cultivate on artificial culture media. The leptospires are an exception, for they will grow in a special serum-enriched medium or in embryonated eggs. The laboratory diagnosis of spirochetal diseases is made by microscopic demonstration of the organisms in appropriate clinical specimens, when possible; in special cultures in the case of leptospirosis; or, most frequently, by serological methods for detecting antibodies in the patient's serum (see Part 4).

Treponema. The most important member of this genus is *Treponema pallidum,* the agent of syphilis. The organism can be demonstrated by dark-field examination of material from the primary lesion of the disease, called a *chancre.* Diagnostic serological tests for syphilis are numerous. They are particularly valuable because syphilis can be a latent, silent infection, with few or no obvious symptoms in its early stages. It is a chronic, progressive disease, however, and if unrecognized and untreated it can have very serious consequences. Also, it is a sexually transmitted disease, highly communicable in its primary stage. Laboratory diagnosis of syphilis is, therefore, essential in its recognition, treatment, and control.

Nonpathogenic species of *Treponema* are frequent members of the normal flora of the mouth and gums, and sometimes of the genital membranes.

Borrelia. *Borrelia* species are pathogenic for humans and a wide variety of animals including rodents, birds, and cattle. They are transmitted by the bites of arthropods. The two most important species for humans are *Borrelia recurrentis,* the agent of relapsing fever, and *Borrelia burgdorferi,* the agent of Lyme disease.

Relapsing fever is now primarily a tropical disease, and is transmitted by lice. As the name implies, the infection is characterized by repeated episodes of fever with afebrile intervals in between. Diagnosis is made primarily by seeing the organisms in the patient's blood either in an unstained preparation viewed by dark-field microscopy or in a smear stained with routine dyes used in the hematology laboratory (e.g., Giemsa stain).

Lyme disease, transmitted by ticks, occurs in a number of countries. In the United States, it was first recognized in children living in Lyme, Connecticut. Although once thought to be confined to the eastern part of the United States, this disease is a growing problem in numerous parts of the country. The first sign of infection is a circular, rash-like lesion that begins at the site of the tick bite. This lesion may remain localized or spread to other body areas. The rash may be accompanied by flu-like or meningitis-like symptoms and, if untreated, many patients develop arthritis, chronic skin lesions, and nervous system abnormalities after many weeks or even years. Because the signs and symptoms mimic those of other infections, the correct diagnosis is often not suspected. Currently, diagnosis is best made by detecting antibodies against the spirochete in the patient's serum but a history of tick bite provides an important clue.

Leptospira. This genus is now classified as having only one species, *Leptospira interrogans.* There are several different serological strains that are pathogenic for animals (dogs, rodents) and one associated with a human disease called *icterohemorrhagia,* or, more simply, leptospirosis. (It is also sometimes called Weil's disease.) The spirochetes infect the liver and kidney producing local hemorrhage and jaundice, hence the clinical term icterohemorrhagia. It can also cause meningitis.

The laboratory diagnosis of leptospirosis can sometimes be made by demonstrating the organism in dark-field preparations of blood or urine specimens (this spirochete is very tightly coiled, its ends are characteristically hooked, and it has a rapid, lashing motility). Culture of such specimens in serum medium (Fletcher's) or animal inoculation can also lead to recovery of the spirochete. Serological diagnosis can be made by testing the patient's serum for leptospiral antibodies.

In this experiment you will see the morphology of some spirochetes in prepared slides and demonstration material.

Purpose	Demonstration of important spirochetes
Materials	Prepared stained slides
	Projection slides, if available

Procedures

Examine the prepared slides. From your observations and/or reading, illustrate the microscopic morphology of each spirochetal genus:

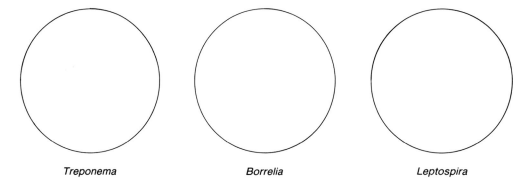

| *Treponema* | *Borrelia* | *Leptospira* |

Questions

1. Can you distinguish between *N. gonorrhoeae* and *N. meningitidis* by Gram stain? Explain.

2. What are intracellular gram-negative diplococci?

3. Why are selective media used for primary culture of specimens from the female urogenital tract?

4. How are pathogenic *Neisseria* identified?

5. Name three agents of bacterial meningitis.

6. When spinal fluid is collected for laboratory diagnosis of meningitis, how should it be transported?

7. Where are *Neisseria* found as normal flora? *Treponema?*

8. Name the etiologic agents of syphilis, Leptospirosis, and Lyme disease.

9. Can *T. pallidum* be demonstrated by Gram stain? If not, what technique would you use?

10. What is the importance of the laboratory diagnosis of syphilis and gonorrhea?

11. Complete the following table:

Organism	Disease	Gram-Stain Reaction	Microscopic Morphology	Laboratory Diagnosis	
				Specimens	Method
N. gonorrhoeae					
N. meningitidis					
T. pallidum					
B. burgdorferi					
L. interrogans					

SECTION 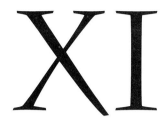 Microbial Pathogens Requiring
Special Laboratory Techniques

In previous exercises, we have studied microbiological techniques for isolating and identifying aerobic or facultatively anaerobic bacteria. In this section we shall see how anaerobic bacteria are cultivated. The general techniques for identifying mycobacteria and microbial pathogens of other types (fungi, viruses, animal parasites) are also described in these exercises.

You should note that these techniques are quite varied. It is therefore important to remember that when specimens are ordered for laboratory diagnosis of microbial disease, the suspected clinical diagnosis should be stated on the request slip so that appropriate laboratory procedures can be instituted promptly.

EXERCISE 28   Anaerobic Bacteria

Reference: Morello, Mizer, Wilson, and Granato, Microbiology in Patient Care, 5th edition, 1994.
Chapters 4, 21, 23.

Obligate (strict) anaerobic bacteria cannot grow in the presence of oxygen; therefore, in the laboratory, media containing reducing agents are used to cultivate anaerobes. Agents such as sodium thioglycollate and cystine remove much of the free oxygen present in liquid media. Cooked meat broth is an excellent medium because it contains many reducing agents as well as nutrients. To ensure complete removal of oxygen from the culture environment, cultures are incubated in an "anaerobic jar."

There are two types of anaerobic jars. One type has a lid fitted with an outlet through which air can be evacuated by a vacuum pump and replaced by an oxygen-free gas. A catalyst in the lid catalyzes the reduction of any traces of oxygen that may remain. The other type is also fitted with a lid containing a catalyst. A foil envelope containing substances that generate hydrogen and CO_2 is placed in the jar with the cultures. The envelope is opened, and 10 ml of tap water is pipetted into it. When the jar is closed (the lid is clamped down tightly), the hydrogen given off combines with oxygen, through the mediation of the catalyst, to form water. The CO_2 helps to support growth of fastidious anaerobes. A second envelope placed in the jar with the first contains a pad soaked with an oxidation-reduction indicator, for example, methylene blue. When the pad is exposed, the color of the dye indicates whether or not oxygen is present in the jar atmosphere; methylene blue is colorless in the absence of oxygen, blue in its presence. Figure 28.1 illustrates one brand of anaerobic jar (GasPak, BBL) in use.

In recent years, improved techniques for anaerobic culture have been developed in response to an increasing interest in the role of anaerobic bacteria as agents of human infections. Anaerobes have been implicated in a wide variety of infections (see table 28.1) from which multiple species of bacteria are recovered in culture, that is, mixed infections.

The ability of anaerobic organisms to grow in and damage body tissues depends on how well the tissues are oxygenated. Any condition that reduces their oxygen supply, making them *anoxic* (without oxygen), provides an excellent environment for the growth of anaerobes. Impairment of local circulation because of a crushing wound, hematoma, or other compression leads to tissue anoxia and sets the stage for contaminating anaerobes, if they are present.

Numerous genera of anaerobic bacteria have been recognized as pathogens, or potential pathogens, and almost all of them are members of the body's normal flora. The significance of their isolation from a clinical specimen may be difficult to determine, and their pathogenicity is not yet fully understood. Generally, they appear to be "pathogens of opportunity"—that is, given the opportunity to gain access to tissue with impaired blood supply, they may grow and cause enough tissue destruction to establish a local infection. The extent of local or systemic damage may be related to a number of factors, including the properties of microorganism(s) involved, the initial site of infection, and the defense mechanisms of the infected individual. Because anaerobes are part of the normal flora of the body, physicians may have difficulty assessing their importance in a culture taken from an infected area. They must consider whether or not a given isolate may be merely a contaminant from the local normal flora as they evaluate a patient's clinical condition. The microbiologist can be of assistance by offering directions for the proper collection and transport of specimens, reporting on the predominance of microorganisms present in a culture, and assuring adequate identification of any significant anaerobes that may be isolated.

Some of the important genera of anaerobic bacteria are listed in table 28.2. It will be seen that the majority of these are either gram-positive or gram-negative, nonsporing bacilli. With regard to pathogenicity, however, that of certain species of clostridia, which are gram-positive *endosporeforming* bacilli, has long been recognized and is best understood. There are many species in the genus *Clostridium*, commonly found in the intestinal tract of humans and animals, as well as in the soil, but three are of particular importance in human disease: *C. perfringens, C. tetani,* and *C. botulinum.* Each of these is associated with a different and characteristic type of clinical disease.

Figure 28.1 A GasPak jar (BBL) for cultures to be incubated anaerobically. The tight-fitting lid contains a catalyst. The large foil envelope has been opened to receive 10 ml of water delivered by a pipette. With the lid clamped in place, hydrogen generated from substances in the large envelope combines with oxygen in the jar's atmosphere. This combination is mediated by the catalyst and forms water, which condenses on the sides of the jar. Carbon dioxide is also given off by the substances within the large envelope, contributing to the support of growth of fastidious organisms. The smaller envelope has also been opened to expose a pad (arrow) soaked in methylene blue, an indicator used to detect the presence or absence of oxygen. When first exposed, the pad was blue in color. Now it is colorless, indicating that there is no free oxygen left in the jar, for the indicator dye loses its color in the absence of oxygen. The jar now contains an anaerobic atmosphere and can be placed in the incubator.

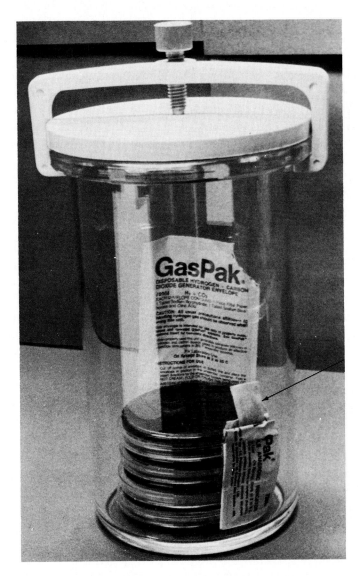

Diagnostic Microbiology in Action

Table 28.1   Infections in which Anaerobic Bacteria Have Been Implicated

Body Area Involved	Type of Infection
Infections of the female genital tract	Endomyometritis Salpingitis Peritonitis Pelvic abscess Vaginal abscess Bartholin's abscess Surgical wound infection
Intraabdominal infections	Peritonitis Visceral abscess Intraperitoneal abscess Retroperitoneal abscess Traumatic or surgical wound infection
Pleuropulmonary infections	Pneumonia Lung abscess Empyema
Miscellaneous infections	Osteomyelitis Cellulitis Arthritis Abscesses Brain abscess Endocarditis Meningitis

Clostridium perfringens is an agent of *gas gangrene* (sometimes in association with other clostridia). If they gain entry into wounded, anaerobic deep tissues, they can multiply rapidly, using tissue carbohydrates, liberating gas, and producing enzymes that cause additional destruction that makes more nutrient available to the bacteria. This can quickly develop into a life-threatening situation if not promptly treated by surgical debridement and aeration of the injured tissue, and by antimicrobial agents. *C. perfringens* grows well on blood agar plates in an anaerobic jar, showing characteristic double zones of hemolysis. Its enzymes attack the proteins and carbohydrates of milk, producing "stormy fermentation" of a milk medium, with clotting and gas formation. It ferments a number of carbohydrates with the production of acid and gas. Usually it does not form endospores in ordinary culture media, nor does it do so when growing in tissues.

Clostridium tetani is the agent of *tetanus,* or "lockjaw." When introduced into deep tissues, this organism produces little or no local damage, but secretes an exotoxin that is absorbed from the area and extends along peripheral motor nerves to the spinal cord. Severe muscle spasm and convulsive contraction of the involved muscles result. It is often difficult to make a laboratory diagnosis of this disease because the site of injury may be closed and healed, with no apparent signs of infection, by the time the symptoms of neurotoxicity begin. The organism is difficult to cultivate, but if isolated, is identified by microscopic morphology and patterns of carbohydrate fermentation. The endospore of *C. tetani* is usually at one end of the bacillus (terminal). It is wider in diameter than the vegetative bacillus, giving the cell the appearance of a "drumstick." The diagnosis is usually based on clinical signs and symptoms.

Clostridium botulinum produces the toxin that causes the deadly form of food poisoning called *botulism.* This is not an infectious, but a toxic disease. If the endospores of this soil organism survive in processed foods that have been canned or vacuum packed, they may multiply in the anaerobic conditions of the container, elaborating their potent exotoxin in the process of growth. If the food is eaten without further cooking (which would destroy the toxin), the toxin is absorbed and botulism results. The disease is difficult to diagnose bacteriologically, but the incriminated food can be tested to demonstrate the toxin's effect in mice, which confirms the diagnosis.

Table 28.2   Some Important Genera of Anaerobic Bacteria

Basic Morphology	Genera	Pathogenicity
Bacilli Gram-positive, endosporeforming	Clostridium	C. perfringens—gas gangrene C. tetani—tetanus C. botulinum—botulism
Gram-positive, nonsporing	Actinomyces	Actinomycosis
	Eubacterium	Infections of female genital tract, intraabdominal infections, endocarditis
	Propionibacterium	Difficult to assess; has had clinical significance in cultures of blood, bone marrow, and spinal fluid
	Bifidobacterium	Occasionally isolated from blood; significance not established
Gram-negative, nonsporing	Bacteroides	Infections of female genital tract, intraabdominal and pleuropulmonary infections; well-established as a pathogen
	Fusobacterium and Prevotella	Same as Bacteroides but less frequent
	Leptotrichia	Found in mixed infections in oral cavity or urogenital areas; significance not established
Cocci Gram-positive	Peptostreptococcus (anaerobic streptococci)	Infections of female genital tract, intraabdominal and pleuropulmonary infections; often found with Bacteroides; established pathogen
Gram-negative	Veillonella	Found in mixed anaerobic oral and pleuropulmonary infections; significance not established

In *infant botulism,* when endospores of the bacillus (endospores in honey have been implicated in a few cases) are ingested by children under one year of age, the endospores germinate in the child's intestinal tract in some instances, and the resulting vegetative cells produce toxin. This type of botulism has been implicated in certain cases of sudden infant death syndrome (SIDS).

In this exercise we shall use species of *Clostridium* to illustrate the general principles of anaerobic culture methods.

Purpose	To learn basic principles of anaerobic bacteriology
Materials	Anaerobic jar Blood agar plates Thioglycollate broth Tubed skim milk Phenol red broths (glucose, lactose) Blood agar plate cultures of *Clostridium perfringens* and *Clostridium histolyticum* Nutrient slant cultures of *Pseudomonas aeruginosa* and *Staphylococcus epidermidis*

Procedures

1. Make a Gram stain of each *Clostridium* culture.
2. Select one of the *Clostridium* cultures and inoculate it on each of two blood agar plates. Label one plate "aerobic," the other "anaerobic."
3. Inoculate a tube of thioglycollate broth with *C. perfringens.* Inoculate a second tube of this medium with *P. aeruginosa,* and a third with *S. epidermidis.*
4. Inoculate a tube of milk with *C. perfringens,* and a second milk tube with *C. histolyticum.*
5. Inoculate each *Clostridium* culture into phenol red glucose and lactose, respectively.
6. Incubate the blood agar plate labeled "aerobic" in air at 35°C for 24 hours.
7. Place all other tubes and plates in the anaerobic jar. (The instructor will demonstrate the method for obtaining an anaerobic atmosphere within the jar.) When it has been set up, the jar is incubated at 35°C for 24 hours. When working with actual clinical specimens, the jar is often not opened until 48 hours, except when *Clostridium* is highly suspected.

Results

1. Indicate the Gram reaction of the *Clostridium* cultures and illustrate their microscopic morphology.

C. perfringens   C. histolyticum

What stain would you use to determine whether these organisms had produced endospores?

_____

Would you expect to find endospores in the blood agar plate culture of a *Clostridium?* _____

Why? _____

2. Examine the thioglycollate broth cultures (do not shake them). On the following figures make a diagram of the distribution of growth in each tube.

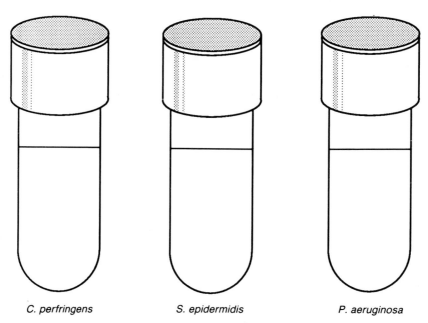

C. perfringens   S. epidermidis   P. aeruginosa

What is your interpretation of the appearance of these tubes?

3. Examine the blood agar plate cultures, milk tubes, and carbohydrate broths. Record your observations:

Name of Organism	Morphology on Aerobic Plate	Morphology on Anaerobic Plate	Hemolysis	Milk	Glucose	Lactose
C. perfringens						
C. histolyticum						

State your interpretation of the appearance of the milk cultures.

Questions

1. Define anaerobe, aerobe, and facultative anaerobe.

2. Describe two methods for obtaining an anaerobic atmosphere for cultures.

3. Can an aerobe be distinguished from an anaerobe in thioglycollate broth? If so, how?

4. If you wanted to culture a wound specimen but couldn't find an anaerobic jar, would a candle jar serve as a suitable substitute? Why?

5. What is a bacterial endospore? Why should it have medical importance?

6. What is an exotoxin?

7. Describe two important properties of *C. perfringens* in culture.

8. Name three diseases caused by anaerobic bacteria.

9. When a specimen from a wound of a patient suspected of having gas gangrene is sent to the laboratory, would an immediate Gram-stain report be of clinical value? Why?

10. If a patient on a surgical unit develops gas gangrene, what hospital precautions, if any, should be taken? Why?

11. What is an opportunistic pathogen (pathogen of opportunity)?

12. Is botulism considered to be an infectious disease? Why?

13. Why should a cook follow home-canning instructions carefully?

EXERCISE 29 Mycobacteria

Reference: Morello, Mizer, Wilson, and Granato, Microbiology in Patient Care, 5th edition, 1994. Chapters 4, 12, 19.

The genus *Mycobacterium* contains many species, a number of which can cause human disease. A few are saprophytic organisms, found in soil and water, and also on human skin and mucous membranes. The two important pathogens in this group are *Mycobacterium tuberculosis,* the agent of tuberculosis, and *Mycobacterium leprae,* the cause of Hansen disease (leprosy). However, *Mycobacterium kansasii* and the *Mycobacterium avium* complex (see table 29.1) cause disease in persons with chronic lung disease and are being seen more frequently as opportunistic pathogens in patients with leukemia and acquired immune deficiency syndrome (AIDS). Table 29.1 summarizes the mycobacteria with respect to the type of disease they may cause.

Laboratory diagnosis of tuberculosis and other mycobacterial infection is made by identifying the organisms in acid-fast smears and in cultures of clinical specimens from any area of the body where infection may be localized. In pulmonary disease, sputum specimens and gastric washings are appropriate, but if the disease is disseminated, the organisms may be found in a variety of areas. Urine, blood, spinal fluid, lymph nodes, or bone marrow may be of diagnostic

Table 29.1 Mycobacteria in Infectious Disease

Disease	Species	Host(s)	Route of Entry
Tuberculosis	Mycobacterium tuberculosis	Human	Respiratory
	M. bovis	Cattle and human	Alimentary (milk)
Pulmonary disease resembling tuberculosis (mycobacterioses)	M. avium*	Fowl and human	Respiratory
	M. intracellulare*	Human	
	M. kansasii	Human	Environmental contacts?
	M. szulgai	Human	(water and soil)
	M. xenopi	Human	
Lymphadenitis (usually cervical)	M. tuberculosis	Human	Respiratory
	M. scrofulaceum	Human	Environmental contacts?
	M. avium complex	Fowl	(water and soil)
		Human	
Skin ulcerations	M. ulcerans	Human	Environmental contacts?
	M. marinum	Fish and human	Aquatic contacts
Soft tissue	M. fortuitum	Human	Environmental contacts?
	M. chelonae	Human	
Hansen disease (leprosy)	M. leprae	Human	Respiratory
Saprophytes: water, soil; human skin and mucosae	M. smegmatis		
	M. phlei		
	M. gordonae		

*Mycobacterium avium and M. intracellulare are so closely related that they are often identified as the Mycobacterium avium complex.

value, especially in immunocompromised patients. Any specimen collected for identification of mycobacteria must be handled with particular caution and strict asepsis. These organisms, with their thick waxy coats, can survive for long periods even under adverse environmental conditions. They can remain viable for long periods in dried sputum or other infectious discharges and they are also resistant to many disinfectants. Choosing a suitable disinfectant for chemical destruction of tubercle bacilli requires careful consideration.

The Kinyoun stain (see Exercise 6) is commonly used to stain acid-fast bacilli. The organisms stain red against a blue background, whereas non-acid-fast organisms are blue (see colorplate 8). Tubercle bacilli are slender rods, often beaded in appearance.

Special media containing complex nutrients, such as eggs, potato, and serum, are used for culture of tubercle bacilli. Lowenstein-Jensen's medium is a solid egg medium used as a slant and is one of several in common use.

Tubercle bacilli and most other mycobacteria grow very slowly. At least several days, and up to four to eight weeks for *M. tuberculosis,* are required for visible growth to appear. They are aerobic organisms, but their growth can be accelerated to some extent with increased atmospheric CO_2. A few biochemical reactions are used to distinguish the colonial growth of *M. tuberculosis* from that of other species.

M. leprae (also known as Hansen bacillus) cannot be cultivated on laboratory media. Laboratory diagnosis of Hansen disease is based only on direct microscopic examination of acid-fast smears of material from the lesions.

EXPERIMENT 29.1   Microscopic Morphology of *Mycobacterium tuberculosis*

Purpose	To study *M. tuberculosis* in smears
Materials	Prepared acid-fast stains

Procedures

Examine the prepared slides under oil immersion. Make a colored drawing of tubercle bacilli as you see them.

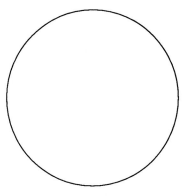

State your interpretation of the term "acid-fast."

Diagnostic Microbiology in Action

EXPERIMENT **29.2**   **Culturing a Sputum Specimen for Mycobacteria**

Purpose	To study mycobacteria in culture
Materials	Lowenstein-Jensen slants
	Simulated sputum culture (predigested and concentrated)

Procedures

1. Prepare an acid-fast stain directly from the sputum specimen (review Exercise 6). Read and record observations.
2. Inoculate the specimen on Lowenstein-Jensen medium and incubate at 35°C until growth appears.
3. Examine for visible growth and record appearance.

Results

1. Diagram observations of the stained smear.

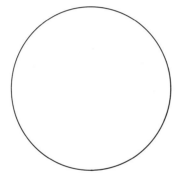

2. Describe the growth on Lowenstein-Jensen medium. How many days before growth appeared?

Questions

1. Name two saprophytic, commensal species of *Mycobacterium*.

2. What is Hansen bacillus?

3. From your reading, can you explain why sputum is "digested" and concentrated prior to culture?

4. Why are tubercle bacilli acid-fast?

5. Why are tubercle bacilli difficult to destroy by chemical disinfection?

6. What special precautions are necessary for collecting and handling specimens from tuberculosis patients?

7. Is the presence of acid-fast bacilli in a sputum sufficient evidence of tuberculosis? Why?

8. Why do some culture reports for pathogenic mycobacteria require 6 or more weeks?

9. If you were caring for a patient with tuberculosis, how often would you wash your hands? With what?

10. In the United States, an acid-fast isolate from an AIDS patient is most likely to be which mycobacterial species?

EXERCISE **30** Mycoplasmas, Rickettsiae, Chlamydiae, and Viruses

Reference: Morello, Mizer, Wilson, and Granato, Microbiology in Patient Care, 5th edition, 1994. Chapters 2, 12, 13, 17, 19, 22.

The first three of these groups are classified as true bacteria, but they are extremely small, and for various reasons not cultivable by ordinary bacteriologic methods. The viruses are the smallest of all microorganisms and are classified separately. The techniques that have developed over many years for propagating and studying viruses have provided an understanding of their nature and pathogenicity. The electron microscope, together with elegantly precise biochemical, physical, molecular, and immunologic procedures, has revealed the structure of viruses and their role in disease at the cellular level.

In this exercise we shall review the nature and pathogenicity of these microorganisms.

Purpose	To learn the role of mycoplasmas, rickettsiae, chlamydiae, and viruses in disease and to review some laboratory procedures for recognizing them
Materials	Projection slides illustrating each group Diagram of the electron microscope

Procedures

Students will not perform laboratory procedures, but should come to class prepared by assigned reading to discuss the laboratory diagnosis of diseases caused by these agents.

Following is a brief summary of each group.

Mycoplasmas

The mycoplasmas, previously called "pleuropneumonia-like organisms" (PPLO), were first known as etiologic agents of bovine pleuropneumonia. Several species are now recognized, including three that are agents of human infectious disease. These are:

Mycoplasma pneumoniae is the causative organism of "atypical primary pneumonia." The term implies that the disease is unlike bacterial pneumonias and does not represent a secondary infection by an opportunistic invader, but has a single primary agent. Clinically, mycoplasmal pneumonia is an influenza-like illness.

Mycoplasma hominis may be found on healthy mucous membranes, but is also associated with some cases of postpartum fever, pyelonephritis, wound infection, and arthritis.

Ureaplasmas are strains of mycoplasma that produce very tiny colonies and were, for this reason, once called "T-mycoplasmas." They have been renamed in recognition of their unique possession of the enzyme urease. These mycoplasmas, like *M. hominis,* are normally found on mucosal surfaces, but have sometimes been associated with urogenital and neonatal infections and female infertility.

Mycoplasmas are extremely pleomorphic (varied in size and shape). They are very thin and plastic because they lack cell walls. For this reason, unlike other bacteria, they can pass through bacterial filters, they do not stain with ordinary dyes, and they are resistant to antimicrobial agents (such as penicillin) that act by interfering with cell wall synthesis.

These organisms can be cultivated on enriched culture media, but on agar media their colonies can be clearly visualized only with magnifying lenses. They do not heap on the surface, but extend into and through the agar from the point of inoculation.

Specimens for laboratory diagnosis include sputum, urethral or cervical discharge, synovial fluid, or any material representative of the site of suspected infection. Cultures require three to ten days of incubation at 35°C. Serological methods are also available for detecting mycoplasmal antibodies in the patient's serum.

Rickettsiae

The rickettsiae are very small bacteria that survive only when growing and multiplying intracellularly in living tissue. In this respect they are like viruses; that is, they are obligate parasites. They have a cell wall similar to that of other bacteria, which can be stained with special stains so that their morphology can be studied with the light microscope. However, in the laboratory they can be propagated only in cell culture or in intact animals, such as chick embryos, mice, and guinea pigs. They are identified by their growth characteristics, by the type of injury they create in cells or animals, and by serological means. Serological diagnosis of rickettsial diseases can also be made by identifying patients' serum antibodies.

Certain arthropods, such as ticks, mites, or lice, are the natural reservoirs of rickettsiae. They are transmitted to humans by the bite of such insects, by rubbing infected insect feces into skin (for example, after a bite), or by inhaling aerosols contaminated by infected insects. The most important rickettsial pathogens are *Rickettsia prowazekii* (epidemic typhus), *Rickettsia rickettsii* (Rocky Mountain spotted fever), *Rickettsia akari* (rickettsialpox), and *Coxiella burnetii* (Q fever). Following is a list of the major groups of rickettsiae and the diseases they cause.

I. Typhus group
   A. Epidemic typhus
   B. Murine typhus
   C. Scrub typhus (tsutsugamushi fever)
II. Spotted fever group
   A. Rocky Mountain spotted fever
   B. Rickettsialpox
   C. Boutonneuse fever
III. Q Fever

Chlamydiae

The chlamydiae are intermediate in size between rickettsiae and the largest viruses, which they were once thought to be. They are now recognized as true bacteria because of the structure and composition of their cell walls (the term chlamydia means "thick-walled") and because their basic reproductive mechanism is of the bacterial type. They are nonmotile, coccoid organisms which, like the rickettsiae, are obligate parasites. Their intracellular life is characterized by a unique developmental cycle. When first taken up by a parasitized cell, the chlamydial organism becomes enveloped within a membranous vacuole. This "elementary body" then reorganizes and enlarges, becoming what is called a "reticulate body." The latter, still within its vacuole, then begins to divide repeatedly by binary fission, producing a mass of small particles termed an "inclusion body" (see colorplate 24). Eventually the particles are freed from the cell, and each of the new small particles (again called elementary bodies) may then infect another cell, beginning the cycle again.

Three chlamydial species are responsible for human disease. *Chlamydia psittaci* causes ornithosis, or psittacosis ("parrot" fever), a pneumonia transmitted to humans usually by certain pet birds. *Chlamydia trachomatis* currently is the most common agent of sexually transmitted disease; the infection is referred to as nongonococcal urethritis. In addition, this species causes a less common sexually transmitted disease, lymphogranuloma venereum; infant pneumonitis; and trachoma, a severe eye disease that can lead to blindness. *Chlamydia pneumoniae* produces a variety of respiratory diseases, especially in young adults. Because of difficulties growing it, the organism was identified only during the 1980s. Undoubtedly it has been causing disease for many years, if not for centuries.

Table 30.1   Clinical and Epidemiological Classification of Some Viruses

Respiratory Viruses	*Poxviruses*	*Arboviruses* (Arthropod-borne)
Influenza virus	(Dermotropic)	(Viscerotropic)
Parainfluenza viruses	Smallpox (variola virus)	Yellow fever virus
Adenoviruses	Cowpox virus	Dengue fever virus
Rhinoviruses	Vaccinia virus	Colorado tick fever virus
Respiratory syncytial		Sandfly fever virus
(RS) virus	*Herpesviruses*	(Neurotropic)
Mumps virus	(Dermotropic and viscerotropic)	Eastern equine encephalitis virus
	Chickenpox (varicella-zoster virus)	Western equine encephalitis virus
Enteric Viruses	Herpes simplex virus, types 1 and 2	St. Louis encephalitis virus
Poliomyelitis virus	Infectious mononucleosis (E-B virus)	Japanese B encephalitis virus
Coxsackie viruses	Cytomegalovirus	
ECHO viruses		*Other*
Hepatitis A virus (infectious)	*Exanthem Viruses*	(Transmitted by blood)
Rotavirus	(Dermotropic and viscerotropic)	Hepatitis B virus (serum)
	Measles (rubeola virus)	Human immunodeficiency viruses
	German measles (rubella virus)	
	CNS Virus	
	(Neurotropic)	
	Rabies virus	

Viruses

Viruses are infectious agents that reproduce only within intact living cells. They are so small and simple in structure, and so limited in almost all activity, that they challenge our definitions of life and of living organisms. The smallest are comparable in size to a large molecule. Structurally, they are not true cells but subunits, containing only an essential nucleic acid wrapped in a protein coat, or *capsid.* The electron microscope reveals that they have various shapes, some being merely globular, others rodlike, and some with a head and tailpiece resembling a tadpole. When viruses are purified, their crystalline forms may have distinctive patterns. An intact, noncrystallized virus particle is called a *virion.*

In the laboratory, viruses can be grown in cell culture, in embryonated eggs, or in experimental animals. They are identified by the kind of pathology (disease or damage) they produce (see colorplate 25) and by serological tests of their antigens. As in other infectious diseases, virus infections cause antibody production in the host, so that serological tests of patients' sera are often useful in diagnosis.

There are many ways to classify viruses, on the basis of their chemical composition, morphology, and similar measurable properties. From the clinical point of view, it seems practical to classify them on the basis of the type of disease they produce. This, in turn, is based on their differing affinities for particular types of host cells or tissues. Thus, we speak of *neurotropic* viruses as those that have a specific affinity for cells of the nervous system. *Dermotropic* viruses affect the epithelial cells of the skin, and *viscerotropic* viruses parasitize internal organs, notably the liver. *Enteric viruses* are so-called because they enter the body through the gastrointestinal tract. Their primary disease effects are exerted elsewhere, however, when they have been disseminated from this site of initial localization. The term *arbovirus* is used for those viruses that exist in arthropod reservoirs and are transmitted to humans by their biting insect hosts (that is, they are *arthropodborne*). Still other viruses, such as the human immunodeficiency virus, have effects on multiple body systems. In table 30.1, some important viruses are grouped in a clinical and epidemiological classification that reflects either their route of transmission or the type of disease they cause in humans.

Questions

1. What are mycoplasmas? How are they identified?

2. Can mycoplasmas be studied with the light microscope? If so, what kind of preparations are made?

3. What are the functions of the bacterial cell wall? How does its absence affect the behavior of bacteria?

4. How do mycoplasmas differ from other bacteria?

5. How do viruses differ from other microorganisms?

6. How are rickettsiae transmitted?

7. Name the important chlamydial diseases.

8. How are viruses identified in the laboratory?

9. What is an arbovirus?

10. Define cell culture.

11. How does the electron microscope differ from the light microscope? Describe its principles.

12. Complete the following table.

Disease	Type of Virus	Major Symptoms	Transmission	Immunization
Rabies				
Poliomyelitis				
Influenza				
Rubella				
Chickenpox				
Shingles (zoster)				
Smallpox				
Mumps				
Infectious hepatitis				
Serum hepatitis				
Dengue				

13. Complete the following table.

Disease	Name of Organism	Transmission to Humans
Rocky Mountain spotted fever		
Epidemic typhus		
Rickettsialpox		
Q fever		
Trachoma		
Psittacosis		

EXERCISE 31 Fungi: Yeasts and Molds

Reference: Morello, Mizer, Wilson, and Granato, Microbiology in Patient Care, 5th edition, 1994. Chapters 2, 14, 19.

Medical mycology is concerned with the study and identification of the pathogenic yeasts and molds, collectively called *fungi* (sing., *fungus*). You should be familiar with a number of important mycotic diseases.

Yeasts are unicellular fungi that reproduce by budding, that is, by forming and pinching off daughter cells (see colorplate 27). Yeast cells are much larger (about five to eight times) than bacterial cells. The best-known (and most useful) species is "bakers' yeast," *Saccharomyces cerevisiae,* used in bread making and in fermentations for wine and beer production.

Molds are multicellular, higher forms of fungi. They are composed of filaments called *hyphae,* abundantly interwoven in a mat called the *mycelium.* Specialized structures for reproduction arise from the hyphae and produce *conidia* (also called *spores*), each of which can germinate to form new growth of the fungus. The visible growth of a mold often has a fuzzy appearance because the mycelium extends upward from its vegetative base of growth, thrusting specialized hyphae that bear conidia into the air. This portion is called the *aerial* mycelium. You have often seen this on moldy bread or other food, and you have probably also noted that different molds vary in color (black, green, yellow) because of their conidial pigment (see colorplate 26).

Most of the thousands of species of yeasts and molds that are found in nature are saprophytic and incapable of causing disease. Indeed, many are extremely useful in the processing of certain foods (such as cheeses) and as a source of antimicrobial agents. *Penicillium notatum,* for example, is the mold that produces penicillin.

Mycotic Diseases and Their Agents

Fungal diseases fall into three clinical patterns: *superficial* infections on surface epithelial structures (skin, hair, nails), *systemic* infections of deep tissues, and *subcutaneous* infections.

Superficial Mycoses

The pathogenic fungi that cause infections of skin, hair, or nails are often referred to collectively as *dermatophytes.* There are three major genera of dermatophytes:

Trichophyton. This genus contains many species (e.g., *T. mentagrophytes, T. rubrum, T. tonsurans*) associated with "ringworm" infections of the scalp, body, nails, and feet. "Athlete's foot" is perhaps the most common of these infections.

Microsporum. There are three common species of this genus: *M. audouini, M. canis,* and *M. gypseum.* These fungi cause ringworm infections of the hair and scalp, and also of the body.

Epidermophyton. One species, *E. floccosum,* causes ringworm of the body, including "athlete's foot." It does not affect hair or nails.

These superficial fungal infections are called ringworm because the lesions are often circular in form. The medical term for ringworm is *tinea,* followed by a word indicating the involved area, e.g., *tinea capitis* (scalp), *tinea corporis* (body), or *tinea pedis* (feet).

Systemic and Subcutaneous Mycoses

Many of the fungi involved in systemic and subcutaneous infections are either yeasts or display *both* a yeast and a mold phase (they are said to be *dimorphic* because of this). The yeast phase of dimorphic fungi grows best at 35 to 37°C, whereas their mold phase grows optimally at a lower (25°C) temperature. The most important pathogenic fungi that cause systemic or subcutaneous disease are shown in table 31.1.

Table 31.1   Classification of Systemic and Subcutaneous Mycoses

Type	Sources	Entry Routes	Primary Infection	Disease	Causative Organism(s)
Primary systemic mycoses	Exogenous	Respiratory or parenteral	Pulmonary or extrapulmonary	*Histoplasmosis*	*Histoplasma capsulatum*
				Coccidioidomycosis	*Coccidioides immitis*
				Blastomycosis (N. American)	*Blastomyces dermatitidis*
				Cryptococcosis	*Cryptococcus neoformans**
				Paracoccidioidomycosis (S. American blastomycosis)	*Paracoccidioides brasiliensis*
Subcutaneous mycoses	Exogenous	Parenteral	Extrapulmonary	*Sporotrichosis*	*Sporothrix schenckii*
				Chromoblastomycosis	*Phialophora, Fonsecaea, Cladosporium, Rhinocladiella* species
		Skin	Subcutaneous	*Mycetoma* (Madura foot)	*Madurella, Pseudallescheria* species and others
Opportunistic mycoses	Endogenous	Skin, mucosae, or gastrointestinal tract	Superficial or disseminated	*Candidiasis*	*Candida albicans* and other species
	Exogenous	Respiratory	Pulmonary	*Aspergillosis*	*Aspergillus fumigatus* and other species
	Exogenous	Respiratory or parenteral	Pulmonary or extrapulmonary	*Zygomycosis*	*Mucor, Rhizopus, Absidia,* and others

*Also a cause of opportunistic mycosis

Opportunistic Mycoses

Under ordinary circumstances, fungi are of low pathogenicity and have little ability to invade the human body. However, when the host's immune defense mechanisms are decreased by illness (leukemias, lymphomas, acquired immune deficiency syndrome) or by drugs (steroids, cancer chemotherapeutics, transplantation drugs), fungi (as well as other microorganisms) find the opportunity to invade and establish disease. Because few antimicrobial agents are available to combat fungal infections, these represent among the most serious opportunistic illnesses and frequently are the direct cause of the patient's death. Some opportunistic fungi, such as the yeasts *Candida* and *Cryptococcus* (see colorplates 27 and 28), are not always associated with immunosuppression, but others, especially species of *Aspergillus* and *Mucor,* infect only "disabled" hosts. Because the latter organisms are also widespread in the environment, health care personnel must be certain that specimens obtained from immunocompromised patients are always collected in sterile containers and in such a manner as to avoid contamination with airborne fungal conidia. The microbiology technologist must also protect culture plates and broths from such contamination so that any molds that grow out are known to come from the patient and not the environment. Some agents of opportunistic fungal infections are listed in table 31.1.

Laboratory Diagnosis

For the laboratory diagnosis of mycotic diseases, the causative fungi may be isolated from a variety of clinical specimens representing the focus of infection (sputum, spinal fluid, pus aspirated from lymph nodes or other lesions, skin scrapings). They can often be visualized in wet mounts of such specimens. Stains are usually not required for these preparations, but potassium hydroxide solution is used to clear away tissue cells and debris, making the fungi more prominent.

Table 31.2   Some Important Pathogenic Fungi

Organisms	Morphological Features	Diseases
Yeasts or yeastlike		
Cryptococcus neoformans	Yeasty soft colonies Encapsulated budding cells	Pneumonia, meningitis, other tissue infections
Candida albicans	Budding cells, pseudomycelium, and chlamydospores	Skin and mucosal infections, sometimes systemic
Systemic fungi		
Histoplasma capsulatum	*In tissues*, intracellular and yeastlike *In culture at 37°C*, a yeast *In culture at room temperature*, a mold with characteristic macroconidia (spores)	Histoplasmosis is primarily a disease of the lungs; may progress through the mononuclear phagocyte system to other organs
Coccidioides immitis	*In tissues*, produces spherules filled with endospores *In culture*, a cottony mold with fragmenting mycelium	Coccidioidomycosis is usually a respiratory disease; may become disseminated and progressive
Blastomyces dermatitidis	*In tissues*, a large thick-walled budding yeast *In culture at 37°C*, a yeast *In culture at room temperature*, a mold	North American blastomycosis is an infection that may involve lungs, skin, or bones
Paracoccidioides brasiliensis	*In tissues*, a large yeast showing multiple budding *In culture at 37°C*, a multiple budding yeast *In culture at room temperature*, a mold	Paracoccidioidomycosis (South American blastomycosis) is a pulmonary disease that may become disseminated to mucocutaneous membranes, lymph nodes, or skin
Subcutaneous fungi		
Sporothrix schenckii	*In tissues*, a small gram-positive, spindle-shaped yeast *In culture at 37°C*, a yeast *In culture at room temperature*, a mold with characteristic spores	Sporotrichosis is a local infection of injured subcutaneous tissues and regional lymph nodes
Cladosporium Fonsecaea Phialophora	*In tissues*, dark, thick-walled septate bodies *In culture*, darkly pigmented molds	Chromoblastomycosis is an infection of skin and lymphatics of the extremities caused by any one of several species
Madurella Pseudallescheria Curvularia and others	*Tissue* and *culture* forms vary with causative fungus	Mycetoma (maduromycosis, madura foot) is an infection of subcutaneous tissues, usually of the foot, caused by any one of several species
Superficial fungi		
Microsporum species Trichophyton species Epidermophyton floccosum	These fungi grow in cultures incubated at room temperature as molds, distinguished by the morphology of their reproductive spores	Ringworm of the scalp, body, feet, or nails

The medium most commonly used for initial isolation of fungi is Sabouraud's dextrose agar. These organisms grow best at room temperature (22 to 25°C), but they are slow to develop on laboratory media, requiring about one to two weeks. *Slide* cultures are useful for visualizing their structures as they develop and identifying them more quickly. This technique consists of mounting a small square of Sabouraud's agar on a sterile glass slide in a sterile petri dish. The agar is inoculated and then covered with a cover glass. A piece of wet cotton is placed in the dish to keep the atmosphere moist and prevent drying of the slide. Dish and slide are incubated at room temperature or in a 25°C incubator. The slide can be viewed directly under the microscope, or the cover glass can be removed, stained, and mounted on a clean slide for viewing.

Fungi are identified by the morphology of their reproductive conidia, mycelial features, and some of their metabolic properties. They grow slowly in culture, producing large colonies whose gross appearance is also helpful in identification. Some are yeasts or yeastlike, and some are "dimorphic" or "diphasic," as mentioned previously. The latter grow as yeasts at 35°C and as molds at 25°C. Table 31.2 shows the outstanding morphological features of some important pathogenic fungi.

In addition to mycological methods, diagnosis of fungal diseases can be made or confirmed by serological methods or, for a few diseases, by skin tests using fungal antigens.

In this exercise you will have prepared slides and demonstration material to study.

Purpose	To observe the microscopic structures of some fungi
Materials	Prepared slides of dermatophytes
	Prepared slides of *Candida albicans*
	Prepared slides of yeast and mold phases of a systemic fungus
	Projection slides if available
	Sabouraud's agar slant culture of *Saccharomyces, Aspergillus, Rhizopus, Penicillium*
	Blood agar plates exposed 3 to 5 days earlier for 30 minutes at home, in class, public transportation, etc.
	Dropper bottles containing lactophenol cotton blue and methylene blue
	Sterile toothpicks with pointed ends

Procedures

1. Examine the prepared slides and make drawings of your observations.
2. Prepare a wet mount of the *Saccharomyces* culture as follows: Place a drop of water or saline in the center of a clean slide. Emulsify a small amount of the yeast growth in this drop. Add a small drop of methylene blue. Drop a cover glass over the area. If excess fluid exudes from the edges of the coverslip, this can be gently absorbed with a tissue. Examine with low- and high-dry objectives and then the oil-immersion lens.
3. Make a Gram stain of the yeast culture.
4. Prepare a wet mount of the *Aspergillus, Rhizopus,* and *Penicillium* growth as follows: Place a drop of lactophenol cotton blue on a clean slide. Gently pick up a portion of a colony with a toothpick. Using the end of a second toothpick, scrape and tease out some of the mycelial growth clinging to the first toothpick into the drop of lactophenol cotton blue. Try to spread as thinly as possible, but don't rip apart the growth or you will not see structural relationships. Discard the toothpicks in disinfectant. Place a cover glass over the area. Examine under the microscope as you did the *Saccharomyces* culture.
5. Repeat the procedure with any molds you see growing on the blood agar plates that you exposed to the environment.
6. Record your results.

Results

1. Draw the spores and hyphae of the dermatophytes you have seen, labeling each by name.

2. Draw a diagram showing all the structures of *Candida albicans*.

3. Draw the microscopic structures you have seen in each phase of a systemic fungus.

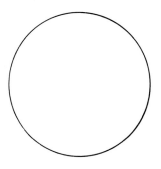

4. Draw *Saccharomyces* cells, indicating any differences in the two slide preparations you made.

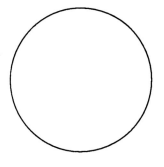   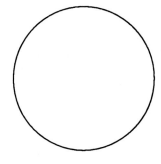

Wet mount, methylene blue   Fixed mount, Gram stain

Color _____   Gram reaction _____

5. List the principal differences you have observed in yeast cells as compared with bacteria.

6. Draw the conidia, conidia-bearing structures, and hyphae of each of the following:

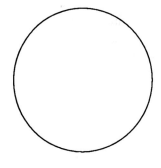

Aspergillus   Rhizopus   Penicillium

Colony color? _____   _____   _____

7. Draw the conidia, conidia-bearing structures, and hyphae of three molds growing on the blood agar plates you exposed to the environment. Do they resemble any of the fungi you observed previously?

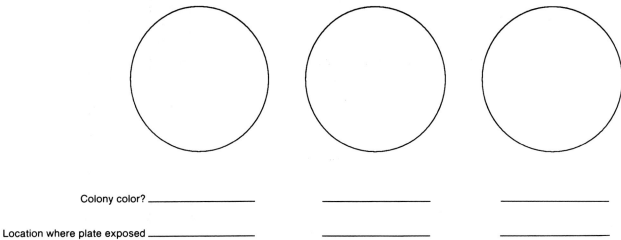

Colony color? _____   _____   _____

Location where plate exposed _____   _____   _____

Questions

1. For each of the diseases listed, indicate the type of specimen(s) that should be collected for laboratory diagnosis.

   Cryptococcosis: _____

   Athlete's foot: _____

   Tinea capitis: _____

   Thrush: _____

   Histoplasmosis: _____

2. What is a superficial mycosis?

3. How would you recognize a patient's ringworm infection? Would you take any special precautions? If so, explain.

4. Should hospitalized patients who share the use of a shower room wear protective slippers when using it? Why?

5. What are some of the valuable uses of saprophytic fungi?

6. How is the Wood's lamp used in the diagnosis of tinea capitis?

7. From what source do patients with *Aspergillus* infections acquire the organism?

EXERCISE 32 Protozoa and Animal Parasites

Reference: Morello, Mizer, Wilson, and Granato, Microbiology in Patient Care, *5th edition, 1994. Chapters 2, 8, 18, 20, 22.*

Medical parasitology is concerned with the study and identification of the pathogenic protozoa and helminths (worms) that cause the parasitic diseases of humans and animals.

Protozoa

Protozoa are the largest of the unicellular true microorganisms. They are classified in the Kingdom *Protista* although their name implies that they were the forerunners of the animal kingdom (*proto* = first; *zoa* = animal).

The basic structures of all protozoa include a *nucleus* well defined by a *nuclear membrane,* lying within *cytoplasm* that is enclosed by a thin outer *cell membrane.* Other specialized structures, such as cilia or flagella (see colorplate 29) for locomotion or a gullet for food intake, vary with different types of protozoa. Four major groups of protozoa are distinguished on the basis of their locomotory structures or their reproductive mechanisms (see fig. 32.1).

Rhizopoda. Simple *amoeboid* forms. Move by bulging and retracting their cytoplasm in any direction.

Ciliophora. Move by rapid beating of *cilia* (fine hairs) that cover the cell membrane.

Zoomastigina. Possess one or more *flagella* that give them a lashing motility.

Apicomplexa. No special structures for locomotion (some immature forms have amoeboid motility). Reproductive cycle includes both immature and mature forms (latter called *sporozoites*).

Species from each of these protozoan groups are associated with human diseases. Some of them are carried into the body through the gastrointestinal tract (in contaminated food or water or by direct fecal contamination of objects placed in the mouth), localize there, and produce diarrhea or dysentery. Others are carried by arthropods, which inject them into the body when they bite. This group of protozoa then infects the blood and other deep tissues. The pathogenic protozoa are summarized in table 32.1.

It should also be noted that some of the intestinal protozoa may live normally in the bowel without causing damage under ordinary circumstances. Some flagellated protozoa frequently are found on the superficial urogenital membranes and sometimes are troublesome when they multiply extensively and irritate local tissues.

Other amoebae live freely in the environment, in soil and water. Under special circumstances, some of these organisms can infect humans. Members of the genus *Naegleria* inhabit freshwater ponds, lakes, and quarries. When people dive or swim in water containing the amoebae, the organisms can be forced up with water through the thin nasal passages, directly into the central nervous system to cause an almost universally fatal meningoencephalitis (affects both meninges and brain). *Acanthamoeba* species are associated with corneal infections in persons whose contact lenses or contact lens care solutions become contaminated by the amoebae. To avoid infection these lenses and care solutions must be kept meticulously clean. Corneal transplant is usually required for patients with *Acanthamoeba* eye infection.

Laboratory diagnosis of protozoan diseases is made by identifying the characteristic structures of the causative organism in specimens from its site of localization (feces, blood, spinal fluid, lymph node tissue, vaginal discharge, or other appropriate material) (see colorplates 29 and 30).

Figure 32.1 Diagrams of four types of protozoa. (a) An active ameba. (b) A ciliated protozoan (*Balantidium coli*). (c), (d), and (e) Three types of flagellated protozoa. (f) Developmental stages of the malarial parasite, a sporozoan (*Plasmodium* species).

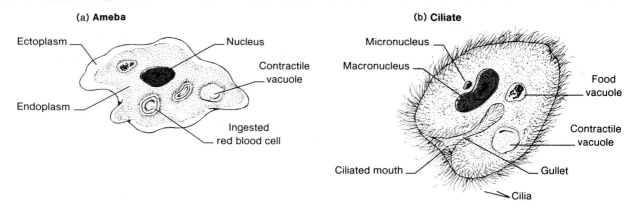

(a) Ameba

Ectoplasm

Nucleus

Contractile vacuole

Endoplasm

Ingested red blood cell

(b) Ciliate

Micronucleus

Macronucleus

Food vacuole

Contractile vacuole

Ciliated mouth

Gullet

Cilia

FLAGELLATED PROTOZOA

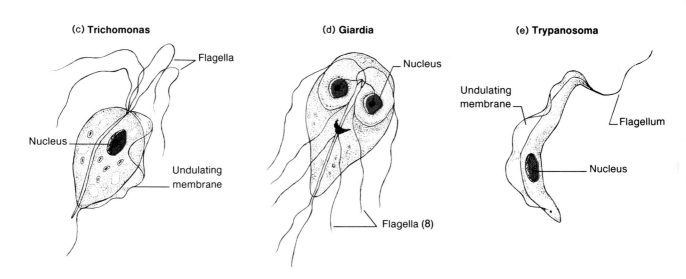

(c) Trichomonas

Flagella

Nucleus

Undulating membrane

(d) Giardia

Nucleus

Flagella (8)

(e) Trypanosoma

Undulating membrane

Flagellum

Nucleus

(f) A Sporozoan. The malarial parasite's life cycle

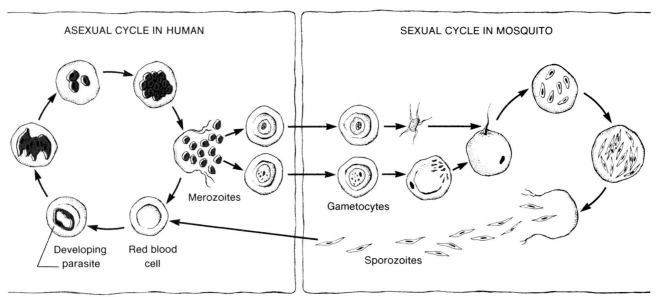

ASEXUAL CYCLE IN HUMAN

SEXUAL CYCLE IN MOSQUITO

Merozoites

Gametocytes

Developing parasite

Red blood cell

Sporozoites

Table 32.1   Pathogenic Protozoa

Disease	Type of Protozoa	Name of Organism	Entry Route
Amebiasis (dysentery)	Amoeba (Rhizopoda)	*Entamoeba histolytica*	Alimentary
Balantidiasis (dysentery)	Ciliate (Ciliophora)	*Balantidium coli*	Alimentary
Giardiasis (diarrhea)	Flagellate (Zoomastigina)	*Giardia lamblia*	Alimentary
Trichomoniasis (vaginitis) (see colorplate 29)	Flagellate (Zoomastigina)	*Trichomonas vaginalis*	Sexual transmission
Trypanosomiasis: African sleeping sickness American form: Chagas disease	Flagellate (Zoomastigina)	*Trypanosoma brucei gambiense* *T. brucei rhodesiense* *T. cruzi*	Arthropod Arthropod
Leishmaniasis: Kala-azar American form: espundia	Flagellate (Zoomastigina)	*Leishmania donovani* *L. braziliensis* *L. mexicana*	Arthropod Arthropod
Malaria (see colorplate 30)	Sporozoan (Apicomplexa)	*Plasmodium vivax* *P. malariae* *P. falciparum*	Arthropod
Toxoplasmosis (systemic infection)	Sporozoan (Apicomplexa)	*Toxoplasma gondii*	Alimentary or congenital

Parasitic Helminths

Helminths, or worms, are soft-bodied invertebrate animals. Their adult forms range in size from a few millimeters to a meter or more in length, but their immature stages (eggs, or *ova,* and *larvae*) are of microscopic dimensions. Relatively few species of helminths are parasitic for humans, but these few are widely distributed. It has been estimated that 30% of the earth's human inhabitants harbor some species of parasitic worm.

There are two major groups of helminths: the *roundworms,* or nematodes, and the *flatworms,* or platyhelminths. The latter are again subdivided into two groups: the *tapeworms* (cestodes) and *flukes* (trematodes). A summary of the major characteristics of these groups follows.

Roundworms (Nematodes).   Roundworms are cylindrical worms with bilateral symmetry. Most species have two sexes, the female being a copious egg producer. These ova hatch into larval forms that go through several stages and finally develop into adults. In some instances, the eggs of these worms are infective for humans when swallowed. In the intestinal tract they develop into adults and produce local symptoms of disease. In other cases, the larval form, developing in soil, is infective when it penetrates the skin and is carried through the body, finding its way finally into the intestinal tract where the adults develop. In the case of *Trichinella* (the agent of trichinosis), the larvae are ingested in infected meat, but penetrate beyond the bowel and become encysted in muscle tissue. One group of roundworms, the *filaria,* are carried by arthropods and enter the body by way of an insect bite. (See table 32.2.)

Flatworms (Platyhelminths).   Flatworms are flattened worms that also show bilateral symmetry. Some are long and segmented (tapeworms); others are short and nonsegmented. Most are hermaphroditic.

Table 32.2   Important Helminths of Humans

Parasite	Transmission	Entry Route
Roundworms		
Enterobius vermicularis (pinworm)	Eggs, via direct fecal contamination	Mouth
Trichuris trichiura (whipworm)	Eggs matured in soil	Mouth
Ascaris lumbricoides	Eggs matured in soil	Mouth
Necator americanus (hookworm)	Larvae matured in soil	Skin
Trichinella spiralis	Larvae in infected pork or other animal	Mouth
Wuchereria and others (filarial worms)	Larvae in arthropod host	Skin
Tapeworms		
Taenia solium (pork tapeworm)	Larvae in infected pork	Mouth
Taenia saginata (beef tapeworm)	Larvae in infected beef	Mouth
Diphyllobothrium latum (fish tapeworm)	Larvae in infected fish	Mouth
Echinococcus granulosus	Eggs in dog feces	Mouth
Blood flukes		
Schistosoma species (see colorplate 31)	Larvae swimming in water	Skin (or mucosa)
Liver fluke		
Clonorchis sinensis	Larvae in marine plants or fish	Mouth
Lung fluke		
Paragonimus westermani	Larvae in infected crustaceans	Mouth
Intestinal fluke		
Fasciolopsis buski	Larvae in marine plants or fish	Mouth

Tapeworms (Cestodes).   Tapeworms are long, ribbonlike flatworms composed of individual segments (*proglottids*), each of which contains both male and female sex organs. The tiny head, or *scolex,* may be equipped with hooklets and suckers for attachment to the intestinal wall. The whole length of the tapeworm, the *strobila,* may have only three or four proglottids or several hundred. Eggs are produced in the proglottids (which are then said to be *gravid*) and are extruded into the bowel lumen. Often the gravid proglottids break away intact and are passed in the feces. All tapeworm infections are acquired through ingestion of an infective immature form, in most cases larvae encysted in animal meat or fish. Usually development into adult forms occurs in the intestinal tract, and the tapeworm remains localized there. In one type of tapeworm infection, echinococcosis, the eggs are ingested, penetrate out of the bowel, and develop into larval forms in the deep tissues.

Flukes (Trematodes).   Some flukes are short, ovoid or leaf-shaped, and hermaphroditic; others are elongate, thin, and bisexual (see colorplate 31). The flukes are not segmented. They are usually grouped according to the site of the body where the adult lives and produces its eggs, i.e., blood, intestinal, liver, and lung flukes. Some of these infections are acquired through the ingestion of larval forms encysted in plant, fish, or animal tissues. In others, a larval form (swimming freely in contaminated water) penetrates the skin and makes its way into deep tissues.

Table 32.2 summarizes the important helminths that cause disease in humans.

Laboratory diagnosis of helminthic diseases is made primarily by demonstrating some form of the parasite in specimens taken from the infected area. Characteristic ova may be found in stool specimens (sometimes larvae); larval forms may be found in blood, or in excised tissue; proglottids or even long sections of tapeworms may be extruded from the bowel. In some instances, serological identification of antibodies in the patient's serum can be helpful in diagnosis, or skin tests using extracts of the parasite may be used.

Prepared slides and demonstration material will be studied in this exercise.

Purpose	To study the microscopic morphology of some protozoa and parasitic helminths, and to learn how parasitic diseases are diagnosed
Materials	Prepared slides of protozoa Prepared slides of helminth adults, eggs, larvae Projection slides if available

Procedures

1. Examine the prepared slides and make drawings of different forms of protozoa and helminths.
2. Review demonstration material and assigned reading on the transmission and localization of parasites and complete the table provided under Questions.

Results

Draw each type of organism listed:

An amoeba:

A ciliated protozoan:

A flagellated protozoan:

A protozoan found in blood:

An adult roundworm:

An adult tapeworm:

A helminth egg:

Questions

1. Complete the following table:

Parasite	Localization in Body (for Helminths, the Adult Form)	Specimens for Laboratory Diagnosis
Entamoeba histolytica		
Trichomonas vaginalis		
Trypanosoma brucei gambiense		
Plasmodium vivax		
Toxoplasma gondii		
Naegleria fowleri		
Enterobius vermicularis		
Ascaris lumbricoides		
Necator americanus		
Trichinella spiralis		
Taenia saginata		
Echinococcus granulosus		
Schistosoma		
Clonorchis sinensis		

2. Describe the basic structures of protozoa. Can these same structures be seen in bacteria, using the light microscope?

3. Are any parasitic diseases directly communicable from person to person? If so, how are they transmitted? What kinds of precautions should be taken in caring for patients with directly transmissible parasitic infections?

4. What is an arthropod? How may it transmit infection to humans?

5. What parasitic forms can be seen in the feces of a patient with hookworm? Tapeworm? Trichinosis? Malaria?

6. What parasitic forms can be seen in the blood of a patient with African sleeping sickness? Filariasis? Amebiasis?

7. What is meant by the "life cycle" of a parasite? What importance does it have to those who take care of patients with parasitic diseases?

8. What precautions should be taken to prevent infection by "free-living" amoebae?

PART FOUR

Serological Procedures

The proteins, carbohydrates, and some other constituents of microbial cells are "antigenic," or "immunogenic," which means that when they infect the human (or animal) body they provoke the production of "antibodies" that react specifically with the microbial antigens. Antibodies are usually present in the circulating blood, where they are a component of serum. When blood is drawn from an infected person or animal and the serum is separated from cells, antibodies in the serum can be shown to react with the antigens that stimulated their production. This type of test is known as a "serological reaction," and the term "serology" refers to such studies of serum for antibody content.

When the nature of the antibody in a given serum sample is known, the serum can be used to identify an unknown microorganism by demonstrating a specific antigen-antibody reaction. You have already seen examples of such antigen-antibody reactions in Exercise 19. Conversely, a known microbial antigen can be used to test a patient's serum sample for the presence of antibody specifically directed against it and thus determine whether the patient is or has been infected with that microorganism. The two exercises of this part demonstrate the principles of identifying microorganisms or antibodies by serological procedures.

EXERCISE 33 Serological Identification of Microorganisms

Reference: Morello, Mizer, Wilson, and Granato, Microbiology in Patient Care, *5th edition, 1994. Chapters 4, 6.*

As you have seen in Exercise 19, rapid and highly specific identification of microorganisms can be obtained by serological techniques. In vitro (that is, outside the body and in an artificial environment such as the test tube), antigens and antibodies react together in certain visible ways. The chemical compositions of antigens differ, and therefore, the reactions are highly specific; that is, each antigen provokes production of a different antibody and that antigen reacts specifically with that antibody only. When it provokes an antibody response, the antigen is known as an immunogen.

In gram-negative bacilli, the carbohydrate antigens within the wall of the organism are called *somatic* (associated with the soma, that is, the body of the cell) or "O" antigens. Each species has a different array of O antigens that can be detected in serological tests. In like manner, those bacilli that are motile also contain characteristic flagellar protein components called "H" antigens (H is from the German word *hauch,* which refers to motility). In streptococci, the carbohydrate wall antigens are used to group the organisms by the alphabetic designations A through V. Many bacteria also contain antigenic carbohydrate capsules that can be used for identification, the primary example being the pneumococci, whose capsules permit them to be differentiated into more than 80 different types. Exotoxins and other protein metabolites of bacterial cells are also antigenic.

The interaction of antibody with antigen may be demonstrated in several ways. In Exercise 19, the latex agglutination, coagglutination, and enzyme-linked assays were described. These tests depend on linking antibody to a particle or an enzyme for a positive reaction to be observed.

The *fluorescent antibody* test is similar to the enzyme immunoassay except that the antibody is linked to a dye that fluoresces when it is viewed microscopically under an ultraviolet light source. Fluorescent antibody tests can provide rapid diagnosis of infections caused by pathogens that are difficult to grow in culture, or that grow slowly. Thus, they have become popular for detecting such organisms as *Legionella pneumophila* (the agent of Legionnaires disease) as shown in colorplate 32, *Bordetella pertussis* (see Exercise 22), *Chlamydia trachomatis* (see Exercise 30), and several viruses, directly in patient specimens. A portion of the specimen dried on a microscope slide is treated with the fluorescent antibody reagent, rinsed to remove unbound antibody, and then viewed under a fluorescence microscope with an ultraviolet light source. In a positive test, bacteria or viral inclusions fluoresce an apple green (see colorplate 32). This test is used in a similar way to identify microorganisms isolated on culture plates or in cell cultures.

A simpler test, which detects O and H antigens of gram-negative enteric bacilli (usually *Salmonella* and *Shigella* species and *Escherichia coli*), is the bacterial agglutination test. When an unknown organism isolated in culture is mixed with an antiserum (prepared in animals) that contains antibodies specific for its antigenic makeup, agglutination (clumping) of the bacteria occurs. If the antiserum does not contain specific antibodies, no clumping is seen. A control test in which saline is substituted for the antiserum must always be included to be certain that the organism does not clump in the absence of the antibodies.

In this exercise, you will see how a microorganism can be identified by an interaction of its surface antigens with a known agglutinin that produces a visible agglutination of the bacterial cells.

Purpose	To illustrate identification of a microorganism by the slide agglutination technique
Materials	Glass slides
	70% alcohol
	Saline (0.85%)
	Pasteur pipettes
	Heat-killed suspension of *E. coli* or *Salmonella*
	E. coli or *Salmonella* antiserum

Procedures

1. Carefully wash a slide in 70% alcohol and let it air dry.
2. Using a glass-marking pencil, draw two circles at opposite ends of the slide.
3. Using a Pasteur pipette, place a drop of saline in one circle. Mark this circle "C," for control.
4. With a fresh Pasteur pipette, place a drop of antiserum in the other circle.
5. Use another Pasteur pipette to add a drop of heat-killed bacterial suspension (this is the antigen) to the material in each circle.
6. Pick up the slide by its edges, with your thumb and forefinger, and rock it gently back and forth for a few seconds.
7. Hold the slide over a good light and observe closely for any change in the appearance of the suspension in the two circles.

Results

1. In the following diagram indicate any visible difference you observed in the suspensions at each end of the slide.

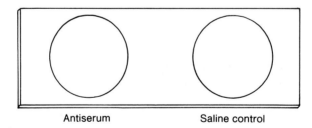

Antiserum   Saline control

2. State your interpretation of the result.

Name _____ Class _____ Date _____

Questions

1. Define immunogen, antigen, and antibody.

2. Name the components of microbial cells that are antigenic (immunogenic).

3. What is the purpose of the control test run in parallel with bacterial agglutination?

4. What is the principle of serological identification of microorganisms?

5. What is the value of serological identification of a microorganism as compared with culture identification?

6. If two separate species of bacteria share the same antigenic chemical group, what would be the result when each is mixed with antibody prepared against one of them?

7. How does a streptococcal latex or coagglutination test (Exercise 19) differ from the bacterial agglutination test that you just performed? What information is derived from each?

8. What is a fluorescent antibody?

EXERCISE 34 Serological Identification of Patients' Antibodies

Reference: Morello, Mizer, Wilson, and Granato, Microbiology in Patient Care, 5th edition, 1994. Chapters 4, 6.

The serology laboratory tests patients' sera to detect specific antibodies. The results of such tests may provide a "serological diagnosis" of an infectious disease in which antibody was produced in specific response to the microbial antigens of the infecting microorganism. Demonstrating increasing quantities of antibody in the serum during the course of disease from its onset (when there may be little or no antibody) and acute stages through convalescence (when large amounts of antibody have been produced) constitutes evidence of current active infection and indicates the nature of the etiologic agent.

The interaction of a patient's antibody with a specific antigen may be demonstrated in one of several ways. Descriptive terms for antibodies refer to the type of visible reaction produced.

Agglutinins are antibodies that produce *agglutination,* a reaction that occurs when bacterial cells or other particles are visibly clumped by antibody combined with antigens on the cell surfaces.

Precipitins are antibodies that produce *precipitation* of soluble antigens (free in solution and unassociated with cells). When antibodies combine with such antigens, the large complexes that result simply precipitate out of solution in visible aggregates.

Complement-fixing antibodies are those that, in combination with their antigens, bind or "fix" complement, a normal component of human or animal serum.

Antitoxins are antibodies produced in response to antigenic toxins. Since toxins are soluble antigens, in vitro interactions with antitoxins are seen as precipitation.

Opsonins are antibodies that coat the surfaces of microorganisms by combining with their surface antigens. This coating on the bacterial cell makes them highly susceptible to phagocytosis by white blood cells. (The word "opsonin" has a Greek root that means "to relish food.")

Serological tests may be performed in vitro (in the test tube) or in vivo (in the body of an animal or human). In in vitro tests, such as those just described, quantitative methods are often employed. An in vivo test may employ experimental animals or cell cultures to demonstrate *neutralization* of an antigen by its antibody. When antibody is first combined with antigen in the test tube, the antigen is neutralized or inactivated (if it is a virus or other microorganism, it cannot infect tissues or cell cultures when combined with antibody; if it is a toxin combined with antitoxin, it is no longer toxic for tissues). If the antigen-antibody complex is injected into an animal, it will not cause disease or damage, whereas a nonimmune control animal injected with the antigen alone will display characteristic symptoms of disease, according to the nature of the antigen. Certain harmful antigens will also be ineffective when injected into animals if specific antibodies have been administered to the animal a short time before (passive immunity). Skin tests constitute another type of in vivo serological test. Depending on the nature of the antigen injected intradermally, a humoral or cellular (delayed hypersensitivity) immune response may be demonstrated. Patients immune to diphtheria experience no reaction at the site of injected diphtheria toxin (Schick test) because their circulating antitoxin neutralizes this antigen. Conversely, when persons who are (or have been) infected by tubercle bacilli are injected with a purified protein derivative of this microorganism, the response is a reddened area of induration at the injection site. This reaction results from vasodilation and infiltration of lymphocytes.

To quantitate antibody in serum, serial dilutions of the serum are made by setting up a row of test tubes, each containing the same measured volume of saline diluent. A measured quantity of serum is added to the first tube and mixed well. The dilution in this tube is noted (1:2, 1:4, 1:10, or whatever). A measured aliquot of this first dilution is then removed and placed in the second tube, containing measured saline. Material in the second tube is mixed, and an aliquot is removed and placed in the third tube. The procedure is repeated down the line of tubes, so that a graded series of serum dilutions is obtained. (This procedure is analogous to preparing antimicrobial dilutions as in Exp. 15.2.) The antigen is then added in a constant volume per tube. After allowing time (at the right temperature) for antigen-antibody combination to occur, the tubes are examined for visible evidence of such combination. The reciprocal of the last (highest) dilution of serum that produces a visible reaction is reported as the *titer* of the serum because it indicates the relative quantity of antibody present. If two sera are compared for reactivity with the same antigen, the one that can be diluted furthest and still show reactivity is said to have the higher titer, that is, the most antibody.

In serological diagnosis of infectious disease, it is almost always necessary to test two samples of the patient's serum: one drawn soon after the onset of symptoms during the acute stage, and another taken 10 to 14 days later. The reason for this is that antibody production takes time to begin and to build up to detectable concentrations during the course of active infection. The first sample may show no antibody, or a low titer that could reflect either past infection or previous vaccination with the microbial antigen in question. If the second sample shows at least a fourfold or greater increase in titer as compared with the first, it is evident that current active infection has induced a rising production of antibody. Such laboratory information is of great value both in diagnosis and in evaluation of the immunologic status of the patient with respect to any antigen tested.

Purpose	To demonstrate techniques for serological identification of patients' antibodies
Materials	Demonstration material

Results

Review demonstration material and your reading assignments; then complete the following table:

Infectious Disease	Name of Skin Test or Serological Test	Interpretation of Positive Result	Interpretation of Negative Result
1.	Weil-Felix		
2. Infectious mononucleosis			
3.	Streptolysin O		
4.	PPD		
5. Diphtheria			
6. *Mycoplasma* pneumonia			
7.	VDRL		
	FTA		
8.	Widal (febrile agglutinins)		
9. Rubella			

Questions

1. Describe a doubling serial dilution of six tubes, beginning with a serum dilution of 1:2 in the first tube.

2. Define serum titer.

3. What are acute and convalescent sera? Why must they both be tested in making a serological diagnosis of infectious disease?

4. Define toxin, antitoxin, and toxoid.

5. Define natural and acquired immunity.

6. What is the difference between an agglutination and a precipitation test?

7. How do immunological tests for detecting microorganisms or their antigens in patient specimens (see Exp. 19.1) differ from serological tests to detect antibodies in patient sera?

8. Why is immunity to tuberculosis detected by a skin test rather than by a test for patient's serum antibodies?

9. What is the RPR test?

10. What is the importance of testing for rubella antibodies in women?

FIVE

Applied (Sanitary) Microbiology

Water supplies, sewage, and food (including milk) are major environmental reservoirs from which infectious diseases are spread. Throughout the world, public health agencies are responsible for controlling such reservoirs and maintaining their purity through the application of microbiological standards. In the following exercises, some simple methods for the bacteriologic analysis of water and milk are described.

EXERCISE 35   Bacteriologic Analysis of Water

Reference: Morello, Mizer, Wilson, and Granato, Microbiology in Patient Care, 5th edition, 1994. Chapters 8, 10, 16.

The principal means through which pathogenic microorganisms reach water supplies is fecal contamination. The most important waterborne diseases are typhoid fever and other salmonelloses, cholera, bacillary and amebic dysentery, and giardiasis. The viral agents of infectious hepatitis and poliomyelitis are fecal organisms and may also be spread in contaminated water.

The method for bacteriologic examination of water is designed to provide an index of fecal contamination. Pathogenic microorganisms do not necessarily multiply in water, and therefore they may be present in small numbers that are difficult to demonstrate in culture. *Escherichia coli,* other coliform bacteria, and enterococci, however, are not only abundant in feces but also usually multiply in water, so that they are present in large, readily detectable numbers if fecal contamination has occurred. Thus, culture demonstration of *E. coli* and enterococci in water indicates a fecal source of the organisms. In water from sources subjected to purification processes (such as reservoirs), the presence of *E. coli* or enterococci may mean that chlorination is inadequate. By bacteriologic standards, water for drinking (i.e., *potable* water) should be free of coliforms and enterococci and contain not more than 10 organisms per milliliter. The term coliform, which refers to lactose-fermenting gram-negative enteric bacilli, is now obsolete except in sanitary bacteriology.

A *presumptive test* for coliforms is performed by inoculating a sample of water into tubes of lactose broth containing Durham tubes. After 24 hours of incubation, the tubes are examined for the presence of acid and gas as an indication of lactose fermentation. Other than coliforms, few organisms found in water can ferment lactose rapidly with production of gas. Gaseous fermentation of lactose within 24 to 48 hours provides presumptive evidence of the presence of coliforms. The test must be confirmed, however, to exclude the possibility that another type of organism provided the positive lactose result.

The *confirmed test* is done by plating a sample of the positive lactose broth culture onto a differential agar medium. Eosin methylene blue (EMB) agar is frequently used. Coliform colonies ferment the lactose of EMB and consequently have a deep purple color with a coppery, metallic sheen. This characteristic appearance of the growth provides confirmation of the presumptive test.

A *completed test* requires inoculation of another lactose broth and an agar slant with isolated colonies from EMB. Gas formation in the lactose broth and microscopic demonstration of gram-negative, nonsporing rods on the agar slant are considered complete evidence of the presence of coliform organisms in the original sample.

Total plate counts are also made of water samples to determine whether they meet the criteria for potability. Instead of performing the broth procedure for the presumptive and confirmed tests, in some public health laboratories a specified volume of water is passed through a cellulose membrane filter that retains bacteria. The filter is placed on an agar medium, such as EMB, the plate is incubated, and then examined for the presence and numbers of coliform colonies growing on the filter. In this way, the presumptive and confirmed tests, as well as the quantitative count are performed simultaneously. The test for the presence of enterococci is performed similarly by filtration.

In this laboratory session you will perform presumptive, confirmed, and completed tests for *E. coli* in water samples.

Purpose	To illustrate procedures for bacteriologic examination of water
Materials	Sample of spring water
	Sample of tap water
	Sterile 1.0-ml pipettes
	Lactose broth with Durham tubes
	Nutrient agar slants
	EMB plates inoculated from a positive presumptive test

Procedures

Note: The entire procedure for the bacteriologic analysis of water requires several days to complete. Therefore, the instructor will provide some material that has been inoculated and incubated in advance to conserve classroom time.

A. Presumptive Test

1. Inoculate 1.0 ml of the sample of tap water into a tube of lactose broth. Label the tube "Tap, Presumptive."
2. Repeat procedure 1 with the spring water sample. Label the tube "Spring, Presumptive."
3. Incubate both tubes at 35°C for 24 to 48 hours.

B. Confirmed and Completed Tests

1. Examine the inoculated EMB plate streaked from a positive presumptive test, noting the color of colonies.
2. Pick a *coliform* type of colony and inoculate it into a tube of lactose broth and onto a nutrient agar slant. Label these tubes "Coliform, Completed."
3. Pick a colony that is *not* of coliform type and inoculate it into a tube of lactose broth and onto a nutrient agar slant. Label these tubes "Noncoliform, Completed."
4. Incubate these cultures at 35°C for 24 to 48 hours.
5. Read all lactose broths for gas formation.
6. Prepare a Gram stain from each agar slant.

Results

Record results of presumptive, confirmed, and completed tests in the following tables.

Presumptive Test	Gas from Lactose (+ or −)	Interpretation
Tap water		
Spring water		

Confirmed Test	Morphology on EMB	Interpretation
Coliform colony		
Noncoliform colony		

Completed Test	Gas from Lactose (+ or −)	Gram Morphology	Interpretation
Coliform colony			
Noncoliform colony			

Questions

1. What is the bacteriologic standard for potable water?

2. Why is bacteriologic analysis of water directed at recognition of coliforms and enterococci rather than isolation of pathogenic bacteria?

3. Define presumptive, confirmed, and completed tests of water.

4. Why must positive presumptive tests of water be confirmed?

5. What is the public health significance of coliform-contaminated water?

6. List at least three waterborne infectious diseases.

EXERCISE 36 Bacteriologic Analysis of Milk

Reference: Morello, Mizer, Wilson, and Granato, Microbiology in Patient Care, *5th edition, 1994.*
Chapters 8, 9, 10, 16.

Milk is normally sterile as secreted by the lactating glands of healthy animals. From that point on, however, it is subjected to contamination from two major sources: (1) the normal flora of the mammary ducts, and (2) flora of the external environment, including the hands of milkers, milking machinery, utensils, and the animal's coat (human skin in the case of the nursing mother).

The bacterial genera most frequently found in mammary ducts are *Streptococcus, Lactobacillus,* and *Micrococcus.* Species of these are most frequently found in milk and have no pathogenic importance. Milk handlers and their equipment may also introduce these and other microorganisms that are equally harmless, except that their activities in milk may spoil its qualities.

Milk is an excellent medium for pathogenic bacteria also and may be a reservoir of infectious disease. Milkborne infections may originate with diseased animals, or with infected human handlers who contaminate milk directly or indirectly. Important *animal* diseases transmitted to human beings through milk are tuberculosis, brucellosis, and yersiniosis. Streptococcal and rickettsial (Q fever) infections of animals are also transmissible through milk.

Human diseases that may become milkborne via infected milk handlers include streptococcal infections, diphtheria, shigellosis, and salmonellosis. (These diseases, as well as staphylococcal food poisoning, can also be transmitted through other foods handled by infected people.)

Pasteurization is a means of processing raw milk, before it is distributed, to assure that it is relatively free of bacteria and safe for human consumption. It is a heat process gentle enough to preserve the physical and nutrient properties of milk, but sufficient to destroy pathogenic microorganisms (with the possible exception of hepatitis virus). The two methods most commonly used for pasteurization of milk are (1) heating at 62.9°C (145°F) for 30 minutes, or (2) heating to 71.6°C (161°F) for a minimum of 15 seconds.

Bacteriologic standards for milk include (1) total colony counts, (2) coliform tests, (3) cultures for pathogens, and (4) testing for the heat-sensitive enzyme *phosphatase,* normally present in raw milk (this enzyme is destroyed by adequate pasteurization and should not be detectable in properly processed milk).

In the laboratory session, you will learn how a total colony count of milk is determined.

Purpose	To illustrate a method for quantitative culture of milk
Materials	Tubes of pasteurized milk diluted 1:10
	Tubes of raw milk diluted 1:10
	Sterile water blanks (9 ml water per tube)
	Sterile tubed agar (9 ml per tube)
	Sterile 5-ml pipettes
	Pipette bulb or other aspiration device
	Sterile petri dishes
	Thermometer

Procedures

1. Review Experiment 15.2 for serial dilution technique.
2. Review Exercise 10, procedure A, for pour-plate technique.
3. Set up a boiling water bath. Place four tubes of nutrient agar in it.
4. You will be assigned a sample of either pasteurized or raw milk, diluted 1:10, from which you will make further serial dilutions as follows:
   a. Using a sterile 5-ml pipette, transfer 1 ml of the 1:10 milk sample into a water blank (9 ml water). Label the tube "1:100" and discard the pipette.
   b. Use a second sterile pipette to transfer 1 ml of the 1:100 milk dilution to another water blank. Label the new dilution "1:1,000" and discard the pipette.
   c. With a third pipette, transfer 1 ml of the 1:1,000 dilution to a water blank, label it "1:10,000," and discard the pipette.
5. Take four sterile petri dishes. Mark the bottom of each, respectively, 1:10, 1:100, 1:1,000, 1:10,000.
6. With a sterile 5-ml pipette, measure 1 ml of the highest milk dilution (1:10,000) and deliver it into the bottom of the petri dish so marked.
7. Using the same pipette, repeat procedure 6 for each diluted milk sample, in descending order of dilution (1:1,000, 1:100, 1:10).
8. If the tubes of agar are melted, remove them from the water bath and place them in a beaker of lukewarm water (about 45°C). Using a thermometer in this cooling water bath, and testing both water and tubes with your hands, make certain the agar has cooled to 45°C.
9. Pour each tube of cooled agar into one of the petri dishes containing a milk dilution. Cover the plate and rotate it gently to assure distribution of the milk in the melted agar.
10. When each poured plate is completely solidified, invert it.
11. Incubate all plates at 35°C for 24 to 48 hours.

Results

1. Count the number of colonies on each plate of your diluted milk sample. For each plate, calculate the number of organisms per milliliter of milk. Average the four figures and report a final plate count.

   a. **1:10 plate:** # colonies $\times$ 1 (ml) $\times$ 10 = _____ organisms/ml

   b. **1:100 plate:** # colonies $\times$ 1 (ml) $\times$ 100 = _____ organisms/ml

   c. **1:1,000 plate:** # colonies $\times$ 1 (ml) $\times$ 1,000 = _____ organisms/ml

   d. **1:10,000 plate:** # colonies $\times$ 1 (ml) $\times$ 10,000 = _____ organisms/ml

   Final plate count = # organisms/ml, 1:10 plate _____ +

   # organisms/ml, 1:100 plate _____ +

   # organisms/ml, 1:1,000 plate _____ +

   # organisms/ml, 1:10,000 plate _____ +

   Total _____ ÷ 4 =

   average plate count _____ organisms/ml

2. From your own results and those of your neighbors, report final results for tested milk samples.

    Pasteurized milk, total plate count _____ organisms/ml

    Raw milk, total plate count _____ organisms/ml
3. State your interpretation of these results in terms of required bacteriologic standards for grade A milk.

Questions

1. Define pasteurization. What is its purpose?

2. Name some bacteria normally found in milk. How can microorganisms spoil milk products?

3. As a bacteriologic medium, how does milk differ from water? How does milk become contaminated with microorganisms?

4. What are the bacteriologic standards for commercial milk?

5. Is it advisable for a patient who is to have a throat culture to avoid drinking milk beforehand? Why?

6. From the public health standpoint, what are the hazards of milk and water contamination?

7. List three milkborne diseases of humans that originate in animals.

8. List three milkborne diseases of humans originating in infected milk handlers.

APPENDICES

I. Notes to Instructors

II. Preparation of Reagents

III. Preparation and Storage of Media

IV. Sources and Maintenance of Stock Cultures

V. Audiovisual (AV) and Source Material

This and the following appendixes contain information that may be of value to the instructor in planning and implementing the experiments.

A complete list of the cultures used in these exercises is furnished in Appendix IV(C). A list of culture sources is provided in Appendix IV(A), and some recommended methods for maintaining stock cultures can be found in Appendix IV(B).

Throughout the exercises, nutrient broth or agar is listed among the materials needed. The most useful media for all classroom purposes are tryptic soy or brain heart infusion agar or broth. When broth cultures are cited for distribution to students, agar slant cultures may be substituted. For antimicrobial susceptibility testing (Exercises 15, 23, and 25), Mueller-Hinton agar plates (commercially available) are preferred, but not essential if the organisms to be tested grow well on the medium in routine use. The following notes on individual exercises may be helpful.

Exercise 1. The Microscope

1. The instructor should carefully review with the student the safety and general laboratory directions on pages 3–5.
2. Each student should be assigned a microscope that he or she can use at each laboratory session.
3. The methylene-blue-stained smear of *C. albicans* may be purchased from the biological supply houses listed in Appendix V(B), or it may be prepared by the instructor.
4. A brief discussion on the metric system is helpful during this period.
5. If other instruments are available, the instructor can set up a demonstration of microscopes other than the light microscope.

Exercise 2. Handling and Examining Cultures

After 24 to 48 hours of incubation, the culture tubes and plates should be removed and refrigerated until the next session. Leaving cultures for extended periods in the incubator dries out the plates and causes overgrowth of colonies, which distorts macroscopic and microscopic morphology. (This applies to all subsequent exercises.)

Exercise 3. Hanging-Drop and Wet-Mount Preparations

1. This exercise should include a brief discussion of flagella and motility.
2. Remind the students to discard the depression slides in a container with disinfectant.
3. A demonstration of motility agar showing a motile and nonmotile organism may be helpful (see also Exp. 17.3).

Exercise 4. Simple Stains

1. Students should be cautioned not to burn the slide during heat fixation.
2. The instructor should explain the principle of fixation and indicate that there are chemical procedures that may be used for fixing microorganisms.
3. Slides should always be discarded in a container with disinfectant.
4. See Appendix V(B) for sources of prepared slides.

Exercise 5. Gram Stain

1. If broth rather than agar cultures are used, the instructor should demonstrate smear preparation from liquid media.
2. If time does not permit full distribution of all organisms, each student may take two or three of the assigned cultures and the simulated specimen.
3. *Streptococcus mitis,* or another member of the viridans group, may be substituted for *Enterococcus faecalis.*
4. The simulated pus specimen should contain at least three different organisms, e.g., gram-positive cocci, gram-positive rods, and gram-negative bacilli. The broths should be heavily inoculated and distributed in 1-ml aliquots.

Exercise 6. Acid-Fast Stain

1. It is advisable to place some old newspapers on the table while applying the carbolfuchsin. This will prevent staining of the table surface if dyes are spilled during the staining process. The simulated sputum specimen should contain *M. phlei* and *S. epidermidis* in about 2 ml of broth.

Exercise 7. Special Stains

1. The instructor should supplement the exercise with a discussion of bacterial structures, including capsules, flagella, and endospores.
2. Instead of having students perform the endospore stain (Experiment 7.1) prepared slides may be examined.
3. If desired the flagella stain discussed on p. 45 may be demonstrated. The method is described in the following article: West, Marcia; Burdash, Nicholas; and Freimuth, Frank. 1977. Simplified silver-plating stain for flagella. *J. Clin. Microbiol.* 6:414–419.
4. See Appendix V(B) for sources of prepared slides.

Exercise 8. Culture Media

The instructor may want to test the quality of the media prepared by the student by inoculating several plates and broths with selected stock cultures.

Exercise 9. Pure Culture Technique

A reliable mixed culture that will yield a good distribution of microorganisms may be made in advance by using a 0.3% sterile aqueous gelatin solution as the holding medium. The instructor should prepare pure cultures of bacteria in separate gelatin solutions and then mix approximately equal amounts. Always use a larger amount of the organism that you are particularly interested in recovering. These suspensions can be held in the refrigerator.

Exercise 10. Pour-Plate and Subculture Techniques

1. The instructor may wish to have students practice pipetting before beginning this exercise.
2. The student should wait until the medium has cooled before inoculating it with the bacterial suspension.

Exercise 11. Culturing Microorganisms from the Environment

1. Students may work in groups in setting up and completing this exercise.
2. The instructor should discuss the importance of microorganisms in the hospital environment.

Exercise 12. Moist and Dry Heat

Experiment 12.1. Moist Heat

1. If each student has two control cultures and two test cultures at one time period, the total is six broths per student.
2. Starch enhances endospore formation, therefore the *B. subtilis* culture can be grown in Mueller-Hinton or other starch-containing broth.

Experiment 12.2. Dry Heat

1. The egg white in the boiling water bath should coagulate in less than thirty seconds. If the dry-heat oven does not have a window for easy viewing, suggest that the students check first for coagulation at approximately the time interval elapsed for coagulation in moist heat, then at thirty-second intervals.
2. The instructor should discuss the correlation between egg white coagulation and that of microbial proteins.

Exercise 13. The Autoclave

1. Sealed ampules containing endospores (Kilit ampules) and endospore strips may be purchased from BBL, Becton Dickinson Microbiology Systems [see Appendix III(C)]. Endospore strips containing *B. stearothermophilus* and *B. subtilis* combined are available from the American Sterilizer Company, Erie, Pa.
2. The *B. subtilis* culture should be grown in starch-containing broth.

Exercise 14. Disinfectants

Experiment 14.1. Evaluation of Chemical Antimicrobial Agents

The material in this experiment is extensive and may be divided among students. The experiment is written for two cultures and one disinfectant solution per student, to be carried through four measured time periods of exposure. Thus, each student, by this plan, has eight agar culture sections to assess, as well as two control sections.

Exercise 15. Antimicrobial Agents (Antimicrobial Susceptibility Testing)

Later experiments (23.3 and 25.3) provide the student an opportunity to acquire more proficiency in performing antimicrobial susceptibility testing, relating the procedure to isolates from clinical specimens.

Experiment 15.1. Agar Disk Diffusion Method

1. The McFarland No. 0.5 turbidity standard is prepared by adding 0.5 ml of 1% barium chloride to 99.5 ml of 1% sulfuric acid (0.36 N). Dispense approximately 5 ml into screw-cap tubes for student use. The height and diameter of these tubes should be approximately the same as the tubes of broth in which the organism suspensions will be made. The McFarland standard is stable for approximately one month after which time the precipitate becomes granular.
2. If desired, antimicrobial disk dispensers can be obtained from BBL and Difco [see Appendix III(C)].
3. A demonstration on the antimicrobial action of dyes can be shown here. A crystal violet solution can be added to a nutrient agar medium, or an assay disk can be soaked in the dye and placed on the surface of a nutrient agar plate. Streak with *S. aureus* or *E. coli*.

Experiment 15.2. Broth Dilution Method

The instructor may prepare the ampicillin broth solution containing 128 μg/ml as directed. Small amounts of pure powder may be obtained by writing directly to the manufacturer (Warner Lambert Co., 201 Tabor Rd., Morris Plains, NJ 07950, and others). One or two ampicillin capsules or tablets can sometimes be purchased from a pharmacy. Alternatively, the students can perform the dilution exercise with antimicrobial-free broth (labeled as though antimicrobial agents were included). During the incubation period the instructor can substitute uninoculated tubes of broth for the higher antimicrobial concentration tubes. In this way a strain of *E. coli* whose MIC falls within the specified range of dilutions is not needed. In addition, the "MIC" can be varied among students to prompt discussion of the experimental error inherent in the dilution procedure.

Experiment 15.3. Bacterial Resistance to Antimicrobial Agents

1. Cefinase disks are available from BBL.
2. Discussion should center on the problem created by hospital-acquired (nosocomial) infections caused by antimicrobial-resistant bacteria, and on the genetic mechanisms for spread of resistance among microorganisms. Tests for beta-lactamase production should be related to clinically important organisms not included in the experiment because of their pathogenicity or fastidious growth requirements (*H. influenzae, N. gonorrhoeae*) or both.
3. Cross-reference should be made to Exercise 18, Activities of Bacterial Enzymes.

Exercise 16. Primary Media for Isolation of Microorganisms

If mannitol salt agar is not available, *Staphylococcus* 110 agar or any nutrient agar containing 7.5% NaCl may be used. MacConkey or desoxycholate agar may be substituted for EMB.

Exercise 17. Some Metabolic Activities of Bacteria

Experiment 17.1. Simple Carbohydrate Fermentations

Students may divide the work, either by culture or by carbohydrate, to reduce the quantity of carbohydrate tubes needed for the entire class.

Experiment 17.3. Production of Indole and Hydrogen Sulfide, and Motility

1. The use of xylene increases the sensitivity of the reaction and is advisable even with Kovac's reagent.
2. A hanging-drop or wet-mount preparation can be set up as a demonstration if time does not permit students to perform this procedure.

Exercise 18. Activities of Bacterial Enzymes

1. The instructor may divide the five experiments of this exercise among five groups of students who can then review all results.
2. Cross-reference should be made to Experiment 15.3.

Experiment 18.1. The Activity of Urease

The urea broth can be obtained in the form of a concentrate (Difco) and diluted according to directions on the tube. With this preparation, there is no need to filter the medium. Students should inoculate their broths heavily and observe the tubes within one-half hour. Purchased slants may be used instead of broths as in colorplate 17.

Experiment 18.2. The Activity of Catalase

The catalase test may also be performed by emulsifying a loopful of culture in 30% hydrogen peroxide on a slide; however, this higher concentration requires greater caution.

Experiment 18.3. The Activity of Gelatinase

1. The X-ray film may be obtained from a hospital microbiology laboratory that uses this method. A local clinic may also be able to provide a sheet of the film.
2. The gelatin tubes may be held in cold running water or in ice water, rather than the refrigerator.

Experiment 18.4. The Activity of Deoxyribonuclease

1. The DNase test can be modified by flooding the medium with 0.1% toluidine blue. Intact DNA stains blue. DNase-producing colonies are surrounded by a pink zone. DNA medium containing toluidine blue is available commercially.
2. It should be pointed out that *S. aureus* and group A beta-hemolytic streptococci are also positive for DNase.

Exercise 19. Streptococci, Pneumococci, and Enterococci

Experiment 19.1. Isolation and Identification of Streptococci

1. The simulated specimen should contain a predominance of group A beta-hemolytic streptococci and some alpha-hemolytic streptococci.
2. The second demonstration plate should show a group A beta-hemolytic streptococcus, a viridans group streptococcus, and *E. faecalis* (nonhemolytic).
3. The third demonstration plate should show a group A beta-hemolytic streptococcus with a bacitracin-A-disk susceptible reaction, and a beta-hemolytic streptococcus of any other group displaying resistance to the A-disk, for example group B. If a

resistant beta-hemolytic strain is not available, you can prepare the plate by streaking both sides confluently with the group A strain. Place an A-disk on one side only and incubate the plate. After the culture has grown, place another A-disk on the other side of the plate. You will then be able to demonstrate a susceptible result and to compare it with the appearance of a resistant result.
4. Specific serotyping reagents are available from Wellcome Reagents Ltd., Beckenham, England (latex agglutination), Pharmacia, Inc., Piscataway, N.J. (coagglutination), as well as other commercial sources. The instructor can prepare extracts for the students or demonstrate the entire procedure.

Experiment 19.3. Identification of Pneumococci

Optochin disks may be purchased from Difco or BBL.

Experiment 19.5. Streptococci in the Normal Flora

Direct detection kits for streptococcal antigen on swabs may be purchased from Hybritech, Inc., San Diego, California or Abbott Laboratories, Abbott Park, Illinois.

Exercise 20. Staphylococci

1. Coagulase plasma may be purchased in dehydrated form from Difco and BBL. Novobiocin disks (5 μg) are also available from these vendors.
2. The instructor should emphasize the importance of methicillin-resistant staphylococci (MRSA) in the hospital environment and their transmission via hands.

Exercise 22. Corynebacteria and *Bordetella*

Experiment 22.2. Bordetella

35-mm slide transparencies are available, as well as prepared slides. See Appendix V(B).

Exercise 23. Clinical Specimens from the Respiratory Tract

Experiment 23.1. Laboratory Diagnosis of a Sore Throat

1. The simulated specimen should contain a predominance of beta-hemolytic *S. aureus* and some alpha-hemolytic streptococci.

2. If the coagulase tests are not positive after 30 minutes, allow them to incubate for several hours until clots are formed and then refrigerate to preserve the clots until the next laboratory session. Once clotted, if plasma is incubated for as long as 24 hours the organism may produce an enzyme (staphylokinase) that liquefies the clot and the reaction appears as a false negative.

Experiment 23.2. Laboratory Diagnosis of Bacterial Pneumonia

The simulated specimen should contain a predominance of *Klebsiella pneumoniae* and some alpha-hemolytic streptococci.

Experiment 23.3. Antimicrobial Susceptibility Test of an Isolate from a Clinical Specimen

1. If *S. aureus* is tested, use penicillin, methicillin (or oxacillin), cephalothin, clindamycin, erythromycin, and tetracycline.
2. If *K. pneumoniae* is tested, use ampicillin, carbenicillin, cephalothin, cefoxitin, tetracycline, and gentamicin.

Exercise 24. The *Enterobacteriaceae* (Enteric Bacilli)

Experiment 24.1. Identification of Pure Cultures of Enterobacteriaceae from the Normal Intestinal Flora

The VP test works best if the broth is incubated for 48 hours rather than 24 hours.

Experiment 24.2. Isolation Techniques for Enteric Pathogens

1. The instructor should use *Salmonella arizonae*. This strain presents less risk for the student.
2. The Moeller formulation of the decarboxylase broths gives the clearest results. It is available from BBL.

Experiment 24.3. Identification Techniques for Enteric Pathogens

See note 1 for Experiment 24.2.

Experiment 24.4. Techniques to Distinguish Nonfermentative Gram-Negative Bacilli from Enterobacteriaceae

A culture of *Alcaligenes faecalis* may be included or used to demonstrate an alkaline reaction in the open tube, which is due to protein hydrolysis rather than carbohydrate degradation.

Experiment 24.5. Rapid Methods for Bacterial Identification

The manufacturers [see Appendix III(C)] of the rapid identification systems described in this experiment provide complete instructions on methods for inoculation and for completion of each test requiring the addition of reagents to demonstrate a reaction. Any pair of enteric bacilli, other than those suggested, may be used.

Exercise 25. Clinical Specimens from the Intestinal Tract

Experiment 25.1. Culturing a Fecal Sample

1. It is not necessary to use both EMB and MacConkey plates. Either is excellent for the basic purpose.
2. In the interest of time and materials, an enrichment broth has been omitted so that subcultures will not have to be performed. Enrichment media and their functions should be discussed, however, and a demonstration should be made of selective and differential plates streaked from an original fecal suspension as compared with those streaked from an incubated enrichment broth culture of the same specimen. Tetrathionate, selenite, or GN broths are generally recommended. The incubation time before subculture may vary among broths.

Exercise 26. Urine Culture Techniques

Experiment 26.2. Quantitative Urine Culture

1. The simulated specimen should contain a pure culture of *E. coli*. This may be prepared in broth, or you may collect some sterile urine and add a suspension of *E. coli*. Refrigerate until used in the laboratory. You can prepare this a few days in advance and get an idea of the actual colony count. If too concentrated, dilute out the specimen.
2. The Quebec colony counter, if available, can be demonstrated.

3. An antimicrobial susceptibility test may be performed on enteric bacilli or other pertinent organisms if any are isolated from students' urine specimens, and if time permits.

Exercise 27. *Neisseria* and Spirochetes

Experiment 27.1. Neisseria

1. The simulated specimen is given to the student as an inoculated chocolate agar plate. The plate should contain a saprophytic *Neisseria* sp. and *E. coli* and be reported negative for *N. gonorrhoeae*.
2. A complete set of 35-mm colored slides on all the *Neisseria* sp. is available from Carolina Biological Supply. See Appendix V(B).
3. Cross-reference should be made to Experiment 15.3, with some discussion of the importance of penicillinase-producing *Neisseria gonorrhoeae* (PPNG).

Experiment 27.2. Spirochetes

1. The instructor should review the principles of dark-field microscopy.
2. A complete set of 35-mm colored slides for *T. pallidum, Leptospira* sp., and *B. recurrentis* is available from Carolina Biological Supply. See Appendix V(B).

Exercise 28. Anaerobic Bacteria

1. The GasPak system, available from BBL, is the simplest and most practical method of obtaining an anaerobic environment. Oxoid (Oxoid, Columbia, Md.) and Difco sell a similar system.
2. If there is a limited number of anaerobic jars, students should work in groups.
3. 35-mm slides of *Clostridium perfringens* showing microscopic and plate morphology and biochemical characteristics are available from Carolina Biological Supply and Color Film Corporation. See Appendix V(B).

Exercise 29. Mycobacteria

1. The student should be directed to review the procedures for the acid-fast stain in Exercise 6.
2. The instructor should discuss the lipid, hydrophobic nature of the surface of the tubercle bacilli and its resistance to antiseptics or disinfectants.

3. The simulated specimen contains *M. phlei* and *S. epidermidis*.
4. It should be pointed out to students that the multiplication of saprophytes isolated in specimens suspected of containing *M. tuberculosis* depletes the medium of nutrient and makes the search for tubercle bacilli very difficult in the mixed specimen. In the clinical laboratory, it is necessary, prior to culture, to digest (decontaminate) such specimens with chemicals or enzymes that destroy bacteria other than *M. tuberculosis*. Fluid specimens are then concentrated by centrifugation and the sediment is inoculated on appropriate culture media.
5. Consult film sources in Appendix V(A) for material on the tubercle bacilli.

Exercise 30. Mycoplasmas, Rickettsiae, Chlamydiae, and Viruses

1. A complete set of slides for projection is available from Color Film Corporation.
2. In answering the questions at the end of the exercise, the student should use the textbook and reference material available in the library. The student should consult Appendix V(C) for source material.

Exercise 31. Fungi: Yeasts and Molds

1. 35-mm slides of a large variety of fungi are available from Color Film Corporation. See Appendix V(B).
2. The students may be given blood agar or Sabouraud agar plates to expose to the environment during the week before this exercise is scheduled. Fungi may require 3 to 5 days to reach a size sufficient to examine. Conidia formation may also require additional time.
3. The formula for lactophenol cotton blue may be found in Appendix II. This reagent is both a stain and a mounting fluid.

Exercise 32. Protozoa and Animal Parasites

1. A complete stock of prepared slides of protozoa and animal parasites, as well as preserved specimens, is available from Carolina Biological Supply. See Appendix V(B).
2. 35-mm slides may be purchased from Carolina Biological Supply. See Appendix V(B).

Part 4. Serological Procedures

1. Cross-reference should be made to Exercise 7 where the capsule-swelling reaction is discussed and to Exercise 19.
2. 35-mm slides of the capsule-swelling reaction are available from Carolina Biological Supply. See Appendix V(B).
3. Consult any of the manuals on clinical microbiology listed in Appendix V(C) for background information on, and the techniques for performing, streptococcal grouping by the Lancefield, coagglutination, and latex agglutination methods.

Exercise 35. Bacteriologic Analysis of Water

1. The simulated spring water sample should contain *E. coli*. The instructor may use tap water inoculated heavily with a pure culture of *E. coli*.
2. In part B, Confirmed and Completed Tests, the EMB plate should contain *E. coli* and *P. aeruginosa*. The student will see lactose-positive and lactose-negative colonies.

Exercise 36. Bacteriologic Analysis of Milk

1. The exercise can be divided so that one student works with the pasteurized sample and another with the raw milk.
2. The raw milk should have added to it a suspension of *E. coli*.

APPENDIX II Preparation of Reagents

The formulae of staining solutions and chemical reagents needed for these exercises are as follows:

A. Staining Solutions

1. Gram Stain (Hucker Modification)

Crystal violet

a. Crystal violet 85% dye   2 gm
   Ethyl alcohol 95%   20 ml
   Mix and dissolve

b. Ammonium oxalate   0.8 gm
   Distilled water   80 ml

Add solution (a) to solution (b). If the crystal violet is too concentrated, solution (a) may be diluted as much as 10 times.

Gram's iodine solution (mordant)

c. Iodine crystals   1 gm
   Potassium iodide   2 gm
   Distilled water   300 ml

Gram's iodine should be stored in a brown bottle; discard when the color begins to fade.

Stock safranin solution

d. Safranin   2.5 gm
   Ethyl alcohol 95%   100 ml

For a working solution, dilute stock solution 1:10 (10 ml of stock safranin to 90 ml distilled water).

2. Acid-Fast Stains

A. Ziehl-Neelsen method

Carbolfuchsin stain

a. Basic fuchsin   0.3 gm
   Ethyl alcohol 95%   10 ml

*For further details on preparation, consult the *Manual of Clinical Microbiology*, 5th edition, edited by Balows et al. (See Appendix V). For sources of materials, see the list of supply houses at the end of Appendix III.

b. Phenol, melted crystals   5 gm
   Distilled water   95 ml

Add solution (a) to solution (b). Mix thoroughly. Filter before use.

Acid alcohol

c. Concentrated
   hydrochloric acid   3 ml
   Ethyl alcohol 95%   100 ml

Methylene blue counterstain

d. Methylene blue   0.3 gm
   Distilled water   100 ml

B. Kinyoun cold stain

Carbolfuchsin stain

a. Basic fuchsin   4 gm
   Phenol crystals   8 gm
   Ethyl alcohol 95%   20 ml

Melt the phenol crystals in a 56°C water bath. Dissolve the basic fuchsin in the alcohol. Add 92 ml of distilled water slowly while shaking the basic fuchsin solution. Add the 8 ml of melted phenol crystals (use a pipette with a rubber bulb) to the stain. Tergitol no. 7 may be added to accelerate the staining of the acid-fast organisms. Add one drop of Tergitol no. 7 to 30 ml of the Kinyoun carbolfuchsin stain.

3. Endospore Stain (Schaeffer-Fulton)

Malachite green solution

a. Malachite green oxalate   5 gm
   Distilled water   100 ml

Dissolve the malachite green in the distilled water

b. **Safranin solution** (prepare as in the Gram stain)

4. Methylene Blue (Loeffler's)

a. Methylene blue   0.3 gm
   Ethyl alcohol 95%   30 ml

b. Potassium hydroxide   0.01 gm
   Distilled water   100 ml

Pour solution (a) into solution (b); mix constantly. Filter before use.

5. *Lactophenol Cotton Blue*

a. Lactic acid	20 ml
Phenol crystals	20 gm
Glycerol (or glycerine)	40 ml
Distilled water	20 ml

b. Cotton blue (Poirrier blue)	0.05 gm

Dissolve phenol in the lactic acid, glycerol, and water by gently heating (20 ml concentrated phenol may be used instead of crystals). Add cotton blue, and mix well. A 1% aqueous solution of cotton blue (2 ml) may be used instead.

B. Chemical Reagents

1. *IMViC Reagents*

Indole reagent (Kovac's)

a. Pure amyl or isoamyl alcohol	150 ml
p-Dimethylaminobenzalde-hyde	10 gm
Concentrated hydrochloric acid	50 ml

Dissolve the p-dimethylaminobenzaldehyde in the alcohol and slowly add the acid. Store in small quantities in the refrigerator, in brown bottles with glass stoppers.

Methyl red indicator

b. Methyl red	0.1 gm
Ethyl alcohol 95%	300 ml
Distilled water	200 ml

Dissolve the methyl red in the alcohol and add the water.

Voges-Proskauer reagent for acetylmethylcarbinol

c. 1. 5% alphanaphthol in absolute ethyl alcohol
2. 40% aqueous potassium hydroxide containing 0.3% creatine

2. *Cytochrome Oxidase Reagent*

0.5% to 1% aqueous di- or tetramethyl-p-phenylenediamine is prepared. The tetra- reagent is stable for a few days in the refrigerator; the di- reagent must be prepared immediately before use and is stable only for a few hours.

APPENDIX III Preparation and Storage of Media

A. Preparation

All media used in the manual are available in dehydrated form. When preparing media, carefully follow the directions on the label.

When rehydrating dehydrated culture media, use only distilled water. Culture media that do not contain agar or gelatin usually dissolve without heating. The exact amount of powdered material is weighed out on a balance and added to one-half the volume of water. Mix thoroughly and add the remainder of the water. When agar is present in the media, the preparation is heated gently over a Bunsen burner flame and stirred frequently with a glass rod, or is dissolved on a heated magnetic stirrer. Bring the solution to a boil to obtain a homogenous solution; allow it to boil for about one minute.

Sterilization should be carried out according to directions on the label. Media containing carbohydrates should not be exposed to autoclave temperatures above 116 to 118°C. Always avoid excessive heating of any media.

Agar media should be cooled to 50°C before pouring to avoid excessive moisture accumulations on the plates.

B. Storage

Preferably, plates should be used on the same day as preparation, but may be stored in the refrigerator in plastic sleeves for a few days. Prepared plates should always be brought to room temperature before inoculation. Always incubate representative plates for sterility.

Bottles of stored dehydrated media should be tightly closed to prevent hydration. If the powder becomes hydrated, discard the bottle. Dehydrated media should be stored in a cool dry place.

Following is a list of common problems in media preparation and their causes.

Table AIII.1 Common Errors in Media Preparation

Problems	Causes
Precipitation	a. Failure to preheat media to ensure melting of agar b. Prolonged heating at high temperatures c. Oversterilization
Darkening of media	a. Inadequate mixing b. Addition of blood when basal medium is too hot c. Storage of media for long periods of time in rehydrated form d. Oversterilization
Decreased gel strength	a. Failure to distribute agar uniformly b. Repeated remelting of media c. Hydrolysis of agar by too frequent or excessive heating
Liquid of condensation on the surface of plated media (leads to swarming, confluent growth of mixed organisms, and contamination)	a. Pouring of plates while medium is too hot b. Failure to dry plates c. Failure to store or incubate plates in inverted position

Table AIII.1 *(Continued)*

Problems	Causes
Inability of medium to support growth	a. Prolonged or improper storage of dehydrated media (excessive humidity, warmth)
	b. Improperly rinsed glassware (may cause chemical inhibition)
	c. Careless weighing of ingredients or failure to include appropriate growth factors
	d. Failure to use distilled or demineralized water
	e. Failure to control pH
	f. Degradation of agar or heat-sensitive nutrients by excessive heating prior to or during sterilization
	g. Prolonged or improper storage of rehydrated media (temperature and humidity not controlled)
Carbohydrate constituents degraded	a. Oversterilization
	b. Improper sterilization*

*Basal media should be heat-sterilized separately from carbohydrate constituents. Carbohydrate solutions may be sterilized separately by filtration or by
autoclaving at: 10 lb; 116°C (240°F) for 10 minutes (minimum).
           or 12 lb; 118°C (245°F) for 10 minutes (maximum).
Taxo carbohydrate disks may also be used if proper controls are employed.

C. Sources of Media

1. Becton Dickinson Microbiology Systems
   P.O. Box 243
   Cockeysville, MD 21030
2. bioMérieux Vitek
   200 Express Street
   Plainview, NY 11803
3. Difco Laboratories
   P.O. Box 331058
   Detroit, MI 48232–7058
4. Organon-Teknika Corp.
   100 Azko Avenue
   Durham, NC 27704
5. Regional Media Labs. (REMEL)
   12076 Santa Fe Drive
   P.O. Box 14428
   Lenexa, KS 66215
6. Roche Diagnostics (Enterotube II)
   340 Kingsland Street
   Nutley, NJ 07438
7. Unipath Co.
   (Oxoid Div.)
   P.O. Box 691
   Ogdensburg, NY 13669

D. Laboratory Supplies

1. Baxter Healthcare Corp.
   1210 Waukegan Road
   McGaw Park, IL 60085
2. Becton-Dickinson Labware
   2 Bridgewater Lane
   Lincoln Park, NJ 07035
3. Bellco Glass, Inc.
   340 Edrudo Road
   P.O. Box B
   Vineland, NJ 08360
4. Carolina Biological Supply
   Burlington, NC 27215
5. Columbia Diagnostics, Inc.
   8001 Research Way
   Springfield, VA 22153
6. Eastman Organic Chemicals
   Rochester, NY 14603
7. Fisher Scientific Company
   Central Offices
   711 Forbes Ave.
   Pittsburgh, PA 15219
8. Pharmacia Diagnostics
   Div. of Pharmacia, Inc.
   800 Centennial Ave.
   Piscataway, NJ 08854
9. Rochester Scientific Company
   15 Jet View Drive
   Rochester, NY 14624
10. VWR Scientific, Inc.
    P.O. Box 1050
    Rochester, NY 14603
11. Ward's Natural Science Establishment, Inc.
    5100 T West Henrietta Road
    P.O. Box 92912
    Rochester, NY 14692–9012
12. Wellcome Diagnostics
    3030 Cornwallis Road
    Research Triangle Park, NC 27709

APPENDIX IV Sources and Maintenance of Stock Cultures

A. Source of Cultures

1. American Type Culture Collection
   12301 Parklawn Drive
   Rockville, MD 20852–1776
2. Bact-Check*
   Bacterial Control Cultures
   Roche Diagnostics
   Division of Hoffman-La Roche, Inc.
   Nutley, NJ 07110
3. Bactrol Disks*
   Difco Laboratories
   Detroit, MI 48201
4. CULTI-LOOPS
   Chrisope Technologies, Inc.
   3941 Ryan St.
   Lake Charles, LA 70605
5. Midwest Culture Service
   1924 North Seventh Street
   Terre Haute, IN 47804
6. University Micro Reference Lab, Inc.
   611 Suite P
   Hammonds Ferry Road
   Linthicum Heights, MD 21090

Clinical microbiology reference laboratories within a local geographic area should be consulted if difficulties arise in obtaining particular bacterial strains. Local hospital laboratories, as well as state or municipal health department laboratories, often can provide advice or assistance in locating sources of stock cultures.

B. Maintenance of Stock Cultures

Stock Cultures

A stock culture may be defined as a standard strain that conforms to typical morphological, biochemical, physiological, and serological characteristics of the species it represents. These strains will possess sufficient stability to display such characteristics reproducibly if they are maintained under proper conditions.

An adequate stock culture collection can be maintained at little expense and requires relatively little time on the part of laboratory personnel.

Two general types of methods for maintaining stocks are in common use:

A. Freeze-drying (lyophilization) or freezing methods requiring special equipment
B. Methods employing appropriate maintenance media held at room temperature, incubator temperature, or under ordinary refrigeration

A.1. Freeze-drying (lyophilization): Organisms in liquid suspension are quick-frozen in dry ice with a solvent and dried under vacuum from the frozen state. Many organisms can be preserved by this technique almost indefinitely. A description of the apparatus and the technique employed in lyophilization is given in Bartlett, R. C. 1974. *Medical microbiology: Quality cost and clinical relevance,* pp. 227–231. New York: John Wiley and Sons.

A.2. Quick-freeze method (recommended for anaerobic as well as aerobic organisms)

a. Grow the culture on an agar plate or slope for 24 hours.
b. Prepare small sterile screw-cap vials. Label each vial with name of organism and date.
c. Add 0.5 ml to 1.0 ml of sterile defibrinated sheep's blood to vials.
d. Remove a generous loopful of the culture and suspend in the blood.
e. Prepare a dry ice bath by crushing dry ice and adding acetone.
f. Place the vials in the ice bath for about 10 seconds. This will rapidly freeze the culture into a solid mass.
g. Store at temperature below −40°C.
h. To reconstitute the culture, place the vial in a 37°C water bath for 1 to 2 minutes. (Do not prolong the thawing time.) Remove a loopful and subculture to an appropriate growth medium. Incubate at optimal temperature.

Most organisms will survive under these conditions for six months or longer.

*Bacterial strains are supplied on water-soluble disks.

B. When deep-freeze refrigeration or lyophilization equipment is not available, a number of alternative procedures can be employed satisfactorily. Appropriate maintenance media must be chosen carefully, in this case, for their ability to maintain the viability of organisms over long periods of time without permitting excessive growth or metabolic activity.

The following media are recommended:

B.1. CTA (cysteine-trypticase agar) without carbohydrates is available commercially. This is a semisolid agar that will support growth for a long period of time *at room temperature.*

Procedure

a. Inoculate a loopful of culture into a tube of broth. Incubate at 35°C for 18 to 24 hours.
b. Inoculate a few drops of the incubated broth into a CTA tube, using a pipette.
c. The stock culture can be maintained from six to nine months at room temperature.
d. Organisms should be checked for viability every two to three months by subculture on appropriate growth media. If sufficient growth is obtained, and if the organism is in good condition, displaying typical characteristics, the CTA stock may be kept further.

If subculture growth is scanty but displays typical characteristics, a transfer should be made from the new culture to a fresh tube of CTA medium.

If the subculture is not in good condition or the growth is atypical, the stock culture should be discarded and a fresh one obtained.

B.2. The more fastidious organisms (pneumococcus, beta-hemolytic and alpha-hemolytic *Streptococcus,* enterococcus, etc.) can be maintained on blood agar slants in screw-cap tubes streaked for heavy growth and kept at refrigerator temperature. These cultures should be transferred once every two weeks to a new blood agar plate for a check on viability and morphology; then to a fresh blood agar slant. Plates may be used instead of slants provided precautions are taken to prevent drying during storage. Plate canisters may be used, or sealed plastic bags. Individual plates should be rimmed with a seal of Scotch tape or Parafilm (American National Can, Greenwich, CT 06836).

B.3. Cooked meat medium (commercially available): an excellent maintenance medium for aerobes and anaerobes. Gram-negative enteric bacteria, including *Shigella, Salmonella,* and *Proteus,* have been known to remain viable for more than five years; staphylococci and corynebacteria have persisted for more than six months. Room temperature is adequate for maintenance.

The stock culture is inoculated into the meat layer of a tube of cooked meat medium. When maintaining anaerobes, first boil the medium to drive off dissolved oxygen; after inoculation, add a layer of about 1 ml of sterile paraffin oil. Although the medium can maintain organisms for very long periods of time, the cultures should be checked for viability every two or three months.

B.4. Ordinary TSA slants with screw caps can be inoculated, covered with a small amount of sterile sheep or horse serum, and frozen at −50°C. In this form organisms are kept viable for long periods of time.

The following special considerations should be kept in mind:

1. Media containing fermentable carbohydrates should be avoided for maintenance of cultures.
2. Selective media should *never* be used.
3. Cultures should not be allowed to dry out; tightly closed screw-cap tubes should be used for storage.
4. *Avoid* refrigeration for temperature-sensitive organisms (*N. gonorrhoeae, N. meningitidis*) although they survive well in the frozen state described in A.2.

C. Complete List of Cultures Used in These Exercises

Acinetobacter anitratus (*Acinetobacter baumanii* is current name)
Alkalescens-Dispar (a teaching substitute for *Shigella* sp. is an *Escherichia* sp.)
Aspergillus sp.
Bacillus subtilis
Candida albicans
Citrobacter diversus
Clostridium histolyticum
Clostridium perfringens
Corynebacterium pseudodiphtheriticum

Corynebacterium xerosis
Enterobacter aerogenes
Enterococcus faecalis
Escherichia coli
Haemophilus influenzae
Haemophilus parainfluenzae
Klebsiella pneumoniae
Mycobacterium phlei
Neisseria flavescens
Neisseria sicca
Penicillium sp.
Proteus vulgaris
Providencia stuartii

Pseudomonas aeruginosa
Rhizopus sp.
Saccharomyces cerevisiae
Salmonella arizonae
Serratia marcescens (pigmented and nonpigmented)
Shigella sonnei (or *Alkalescens-Dispar*)
Staphylococcus aureus
Staphylococcus epidermidis
Staphylococcus saprophyticus
Streptococcus pyogenes (group A, beta-hemolytic)
Streptococcus agalactiae (group B, beta-hemolytic)
Streptococcus mitis or other viridans group *Streptococcus*
Streptococcus pneumoniae

APPENDIX V

Audiovisual (AV) and Source Material

A. Films (F), Filmstrips (FS), Slides (S), Tapes (T), Cassettes (C), Videocassettes (V)

Following is a list of AV sources that may be used to supplement laboratory and lecture material. Catalogs are available on request from each source.

Addresses of AV Sources: *CODE:*

American Journal of Nursing Company   AJNC
Educational Services Division CAT 86
555 W. 57th Street
New York, NY 10019–2961

American Society for Microbiology   ASM
AV/MD Marketing, Inc.
Department MIC-MB 2/86
235 Park Avenue South
New York, NY 10003

American Society of Clinical Pathologists   ACP
2100 W. Harrison Street
Chicago, IL 60612

Boston University   BU
Krasker Memorial Film/Video Library
565 Commonwealth Avenue
Boston, MA 02215

Career Aids   CA
20417 Nordhoff Street
Department AN
Chatsworth, CA 91311

Carle Medical Communications   CMC
110 West Main Street
Urbana, IL 61801–2700

Carolina Biological Supply Company   CBSC
Burlington, NC 27215

Concept Media   ConM
P.O. Box 19542
Irvine, CA 92713

Davis and Geck   D&G
American Cyanamid Co.
Surgical Film Video Library
1 Caspar Street
Danbury, CT 06810

Filmakers Library   FLib
124 E. 40th Street
Suite 901
New York, NY 10016

Human Relations Media   HRM
Room HC 9
175 Tompkins Avenue
Pleasantville, NY 10570

International Film Bureau   IFB
332 S. Michigan Avenue
Chicago, IL 60604–4382

Light Video Television   LVT
21 Highland Circle
Needham Heights, MA 02194

Merck, Sharpe, and Dohme   MSD
Health Information Services
West Point, PA 19486

Modern Talking Picture Service   MTPS
5000 Park Street North
St. Petersburg, FL 33709

National Audiovisual Center   NAVC
National Archives and Records
Administration
Customer Services Section PZ
8700 Edgeworth Drive
Capitol Heights, MD 20743–3701

Software Telemarketer   WCB
Wm. C. Brown Publishers
2460 Kerper Blvd.
Dubuque, IA 52001

Telstor Production   TP
366 N. Prior Ave.
St. Paul, MN 55104

Title	Format	Time (min)	Source	Exercise
The Microscope				
The Care and Use of the Microscope	V		ASM	1
Darkfield Microscope: The Microscope, Part I	F	15	NAVC	1
Darkfield Microscopy: Collecting and Examining Specimens, Part II	F	14	NAVC	1
Journey into the Microscope	FS/C		HRM	1
Microscope	F	11	BU	1
Microscope: Making it Big	F	28	FLib	1
	V			
Using a Compound Microscope	V	14	CBSC	1
The Microbial World Defined				
Amoebae: Single-cell Organisms	F	14	BU	32
Anatomy of Bacteria I, II, III	V	30	TP	4, 5, 6, 7
Bacterial Sporulation	S/T	22	ASM	7
The Bacterial Spore: Dormancy and Germination	S/T	26	ASM	7
The Bacterial Cell: Structure Part I	S/T	11	ASM	3, 4
The Bacterial Cell: Function Part 2	S/T	12	ASM	3, 4
Bacterial Motility	V	16	ASM	3
Between the Living and Nonliving	F	29	BU	30
Fundamentals of Microbiology (Four Parts)				
Part 1. Microbial cell structure	S/T	24	ASM	3, 4
Part 2. Carbohydrate metabolism and energy production	S/T	28	ASM	17
Part 3. Metabolism of nitrogenous compounds. Assimilation of inorganic nitrogen and general reactions of amino acids	S/T	28	ASM	17
Part 4. Metabolism of nitrogenous compounds. Biosynthesis of amino acids, purines, pyrimidines	S/T	33	ASM	17
The Fungi (Four Parts)				
Part 1. Understanding the fungi	S/T	20	ASM	31
Part 2. Important fungal groups	S/T	20	ASM	31
Part 3. Understanding the Fungi Imperfecti	S/T	22	ASM	31
Part 4. Fungal morphology	S/T	22	ASM	31
Genetic Engineering: Prospects for the Future (Three Parts)				
Part 1. The new era of biotechnology	FS/C		HRM	
Part 2. Putting microbes to work	FS/C		HRM	
Part 3. Promise and danger of genetic engineering	FS/C		HRM	
Hookworm	F	10	NAVC	32
Host-Parasite Relationships	S		NAVC	
How a Virus Kills	F	29	BU	30
Introduction to Bacteria	S/FS		WCB	4, 5, 6, 7
Introduction to the Bacteria	V	20	CBSC	3, 4
Introduction to Viruses	S/FS		WCB	30
Life of the Molds	F	21	BU	31
Microbial Genetics Learning Series (Ten Parts)				
Part 1. An introduction to microbial genetics	S/T	28	ASM	
Part 2. An introduction to microbial genetics (cont/d)	S/T	30	ASM	
Part 3. DNA structure and replication	S/T	34	ASM	
Part 4. RNA and protein synthesis	S/T	33	ASM	
Part 5. Bacterial conjugation	S/T	33	ASM	
Part 6. Bacterial viruses, lysogeny, and transduction	S/T	34	ASM	

Title	Format	Time (min)	Source	Exercise
Part 7. Bacterial transformation, recombination, and genetic mapping	S/T	30	ASM	
Part 8. Mutations and the action of mutagens	S/T	32	ASM	
Part 9. Genetic fine structure and colinearity	S/T	32	ASM	
Part 10. Genetic regulation in bacteria	S/T	33	ASM	
The Nitrogen Cycle	S/FS		WCB	17, 18
Parasitism (parasitic flatworms)	F	17	BU	32
Pathogenic Mycoplasma	S/T	30	ASM	30
Protist Kingdom	F	13	BU	1, 2
Protozoa: Structure and Life Functions	F	16	BU	32
Viruses: The Mysterious Enemy (Two Parts)				
Part 1. Probing the nature of life	FS/C		HRM	30
Part 2. Agents of disease	FS/C		HRM	30
The Wonders of the Cell: A Living Factory (Three Parts)				
Part 1. Units of life	FS/S		HRM	3, 4
Part 2. Inside the cell	FS/S		HRM	3, 4
Part 3. Control, reproduction, and development	FS/S		HRM	3, 4
Laboratory Tools and Techniques				
Basic Microbiology Techniques (Series)				
The Making and Sterilization of an Inoculating Loop	V	7	ASM	3
The Development of Aseptic Technique	V	9	ASM	1
Pure Culture Techniques	V	16	ASM	9
Fermentation Techniques	V	20	ASM	17
Miscellaneous Biochemical Tests	V	15	ASM	17, 18
IMViC Reactions	V	14	ASM	24
Testing of Antimicrobial Agents	V	13	ASM	15
Coagulase and Antibody Reactions	V	16	ASM	20, 34
Water Analysis	V	32	ASM	35
Laboratory Skills. Unit 5	S		NAVC	1, 2
Microbiological Techniques	V	16	CBSC	1, 2, 3
Nobody's Immune	F	29	NAVC	1, 2, 3
Preparing and Using Microscope Slides	V	14	CBSC	2
Preparation of a Culture Medium	F	14	NAVC	8
Preparation and Staining of Fecal Smears for Parasitological Examination	F	8	NAVC	32
Rabies: Fluorescent Antibody Staining	F	8	NAVC	30, 33
Staining Techniques	V	34	ASM	4, 5, 6, 7
What is Microbiology?	V S/C		WCB	1
Ziehl-Neelsen Staining Procedure	V	6	NAVC	6
Host and Microbe in Health and Disease				
Anaphylactic Hypersensitivity	S/C		WCB	33, 34
Antigens and Immunogens	S/C		WCB	33, 34
Antigen-Antibody Reactions	S/C		WCB	33, 34
Basic Concepts of Immunology	V	35	ASCP	19, 33, 34
The Body against Disease (Three Parts)				
Part 1. Disease and defenses	V		HRM	33, 34
Part 2. Immune response	V		HRM	34
Part 3. The body against itself	V		HRM	33, 34
Cellular Immunity and Immune Deficiency Diseases	V	30	ASCP	33, 34
Fight Against Microbes	V	29	IFB	33, 34
A Gift, an Obligation	F	28	MSD	33, 34
Hyper-immunoglobulinemias	S/C		WCB	
Immune Complexes and Disease	S/C	23	NAVC	33, 34
Immune Complex Diseases	S/C		WCB	33, 34

Title	Format	Time (min)	Source	Exercise
Immunologic Deficiency States	S/C		WCB	33, 34
Immunoglobulin Structure and Function	S/C		WCB	33, 34
Immunology of Venereal Disease	V	34	NAVC	27
Infection and Immunity	F	14	BU	33, 34
Infectious Diseases and Man-Made Defenses	F	11	BU	33, 34
Inflammation	S/C	25	NAVC	19, 20, 33, 34
The Inflammatory Reaction	F	26	D&G	19, 20, 33, 34
Lymphocyte-mediated Hypersensitivity	S/C		WCB	33, 34
Mounting Immune Responses	S/C		WCB	33, 34
Secret of the White Cell	F	30	BU	26
Prevention and Control of Infectious Disease				
Breaking the Chain of Cross Infection	V	17	D&G	12, 13, 14
Control of Bacterial Cross Infection in Surgical Patients	F	18	D&G	
Controlling Transmission of Infection	V	28	AJNC	12, 13, 14
Disinfection of the Skin	V	23	D&G	14
Disinfection. The War against Infection	V	19	AJNC	14
Fundamentals of Aseptic Technique	V		D&G	12, 13, 14
Hospital Sepsis	F	23	D&G	12, 13, 14, 15, 20
Infection Control (Four Parts)				
Part 1. Basic principles of infection control	S/T	13	AJNC	12, 13, 14
Part 2. Preventing nosocomial infections	S/T	13	AJNC	12, 13, 14, 15
Part 3. General principles of isolation and precautions	S/T	18	AJNC	12, 13, 14
Part 4. Specific isolation procedures for nurses	S/T	9	AJNC	12, 13, 14
Infection Control: An AIDS Update	V	15	CMC	12, 13, 14
Preventing and Managing Infection				
Part 1	V	19	ConM	12, 13, 14
Part 2	V	20	ConM	12, 13, 14
Sterilization Technique (Five Parts)				
Part 1. Introduction to sterilization	FS		CA	13
Part 2. The sterile technique	FS		CA	13
Part 3. Cleaning and wrapping for autoclaving	FS		CA	13
Part 4. Loading and operating the autoclave	FS		CA	13
Part 5. The asepsis handwash	FS		CA	14
Using the Gravity Displacement Steam Autoclave in the Biomedical Laboratory	V	20	NAVC	13
Communicable Disease Control in the Community				
Always Pure	F/V	17	MTPS	35
Food Safety Sanitation	S		NAVC	36
How Disease Travels	F	10	NAVC	
Rabies Control in the Community	F	11	NAVC	
A Safer Place to Eat	F	15	NAVC	36
Water—Friend or Enemy	F	10	NAVC	35
Water Purification	V	9	NAVC	35
Epidemiology of Infectious Diseases				
The ABC's of Salmonella	S		NAVC	24
AIDS: A Nursing Perspective (Part 1)	V	28	AJNC	30
AIDS: Can I Get It?	V	55	LVT	30
AIDS: What Everyone Needs to Know	V/F	18	BU	30
Beyond Fear: The Virus	F	22	MTPS (Amer. Red Cross)	30

Title	Format	Time (min)	Source	Exercise
Chlamydia	S		NAVC	30
Cholera Today: Practical Laboratory Diagnosis	F	18	NAVC	24
Clinical Rabies in Animals	F	13	NAVC	
An Epidemic of Histoplasmosis	F	17	NAVC	31
Epidemiology of Salmonellosis in Man and Animals	F	15	NAVC	24
Erythrocytic Stages of *Plasmodium vivax*	F	4	NAVC	32
Filariasis	F	25	NAVC	32
Herpes Genital Infection	S		NAVC	30
Herpes: It's No Laughing Matter	V/F	20	BU	30
Hookworm	F	10	NAVC	32
How a Virus Kills	F	29	BU	30
Insects as Carriers of Disease	F	10	NAVC	32
Jennifer: A Revealing Story about Genital Herpes	F	28	NAVC	30
Leptospirosis	F	16	NAVC	27
Meningitis	V	20	NAVC	19, 21, 27
Minor Venereal Diseases	S		NAVC	27
An Outbreak of Salmonella Infection	F	14	NAVC	24
Parasitism: Parasitic Flatworms	F	17	NAVC	32
Poultry Zoonoses	S/C	28	NAVC	32
Rabies Control in the Community	F	11	NAVC	
The Return of Count Spirochete	F	21	NAVC	27
The Search for the AIDS Virus: Interview with Dr. Robert Gallo	V	28	CBSC	30
Survey of Sexually Transmitted Diseases by Nurses	S		NAVC	27
Syphilis	S		NAVC	27
Syphilis: A Synopsis	S		NAVC	27
Tsetse: The Fly That Would Be King	F	28	NAVC	32
What Is a Disease?	F	11	NAVC	1, 2, 3, 4
V.D.: A Plague On Our House	F	55	NAVC	27
V.D.: It Is Your Problem	V	14	NAVC	27
V.D.: Photomicrographic Slides	S		NAVC	27
The Winged Scourge	F	10	NAVC	32
Zoonoses of the Agricultural Environment	S	29	NAVC	32

B. Slides for Projection and Prepared Slides for Microscopic Observation

American Society for Microbiology
AV/MD, Inc.
Dept. MIC
235 Park Avenue South
New York, NY 10003

Carolina Biological Supply
Burlington, NC 27215

Color Film Corporation
777 Washington Blvd.
Stamford, CT 06901

Turtox
P.O. Box 266
Palos Heights, IL 60463

Ward's Natural Science Establishment, Inc.
5100T W. Henrietta Road
P.O. Box 92192
Rochester, NY 14692–9012

C. Selected Literature

American Hospital Formulary Service. 1990. *Drug information 90.* American Society of Hospital Pharmacies, Bethesda, MD.

Approved Standard. 1992. *Performance standards for antimicrobial susceptibility testing.* Fourth Informational Supplement (M100–S4). National Committee for Clinical Laboratory Standards, Villanova, PA.

Balows, A., et al. (ed.). 1991. *Manual of clinical microbiology.* 5th ed. American Society for Microbiology, Washington, D.C.

Balows, A., W. J. Hausler, and E. H. Lennette. (eds.). 1988. *Laboratory diagnosis of infectious diseases, principles and practice. Vol. 1. Bacterial, mycotic and parasitic diseases.* Springer Verlag, New York, NY.

Beaver, P. C. and R. C. Jung. (eds.). 1985. *Animal agents and vectors of human disease.* 5th ed. Lea & Febiger, Philadelphia, PA.

Beneke, E. S. 1984. *Human mycoses.* Upjohn, Kalamazoo, MI.

Benenson, A. S. (ed.). 1990. *Control of communicable diseases in man.* 15th ed. American Public Health Association, Washington, D.C.

Bennett, J. V. and P. S. Brachman. 1985. *Hospital infections.* 2nd ed. Little Brown, Boston, MA.

Block, S. S. (ed.). 1991. *Disinfection, sterilization and preservation.* 4th ed. Lea & Febiger, Philadelphia, PA.

Bottone, E. J., R. Girolami, and J. M. Stamm. (eds.). 1984. *Schneierson's atlas of diagnostic microbiology.* 9th ed. Abbott Laboratories, No. Chicago, IL.

Coleman, R. M., F. M. Lombard, R. E. Sicard, and N. J. Renicricca. 1986. *Fundamental immunology.* Wm. C. Brown, Dubuque, IA.

Evans, A. S. (ed.). 1989. *Viral infections of humans: Epidemiology and control.* 3rd ed. Plenum, New York, NY.

Fessia, S., P. Fawcett, C. MacVaugh, and S. Ryan. 1988. *Diagnostic clinical microbiology: A benchtop perspective.* W. B. Saunders, Philadelphia, PA.

Finegold, S. M. and E. J. Baron. 1990. *Bailey and Scott's diagnostic microbiology.* 8th ed. C. V. Mosby, St. Louis, MO.

Finegold, S. M. and V. L. Sutter. 1989. *Anaerobic infections.* 8th ed. Upjohn, Kalamazoo, MI.

Garcia, L. S. and D. A. Bruckner. 1993. *Diagnostic medical parasitology.* 2nd ed. American Society for Microbiology, Washington, D.C.

Gerhard, P., R. G. E. Murray, R. N. Costilow, E. W. Nester, W. A. Wood, N. R. Krieg, and G. B. Phillips. (eds.). 1981. *Manual of methods for general bacteriology.* American Society for Microbiology, Washington, D.C.

Hazen, E. L., M. A. Gordon, and F. C. Reed. 1970. *Laboratory identification of pathogenic fungi simplified.* 3rd ed. Charles C Thomas, Springfield, IL.

Heldeman, W. H. 1984. *Essentials of immunology.* Elsevier, New York, NY.

Hoeprich, P. D. and M. C. Jordan. (eds.). 1989. *Infectious diseases.* 4th ed. Harper & Row, New York, NY.

Hubbert, W. T., W. F. McCulloch, and P. R. Schnurrenberg. (eds.). 1975. *Diseases transmitted from animals to man.* 6th ed. Charles C Thomas, Springfield, IL.

Jawetz, E., J. Melnick, E. Adelberg, G. Brooks, J. Butel, and L. Orenstein. 1989. *Medical microbiology.* 18th ed. Appleton & Lange, Norwalk, CT.

Kee, J. L. 1991. *Laboratory and diagnostic tests with nursing implications.* 3rd ed. Appleton & Lange, East Norwalk, CT.

Kirsop, B. and J. J. Snell. 1984. *Maintenance of microorganisms: A manual of laboratory methods.* Academic Press, San Diego, CA.

Klainer, A. S. and I. Geis. 1973. *Agents of bacterial diseases.* Harper & Row, Hagerstown, MD.

Koneman, E. W., S. D. Allen, W. M. Janda, P. C. Schreckenberger, and W. C. Winn. 1992. *Color atlas and textbook of diagnostic microbiology.* J. B. Lippincott, Philadelphia, PA.

Larone, D. 1993. *Medically important fungi, a guide to identification.* 2nd. ed. American Society for Microbiology, Washington, D.C.

Lennette, E. H., P. Halonen, and F. A. Murphy. (eds.). 1988. *Laboratory diagnosis of infectious diseases: Principles and practice. Vol. II. Viral, rickettsial and chlamydial diseases.* Springer Verlag, New York, NY.

MacFadden, J. F. 1980. *Biochemical tests for identification of medical bacteria.* 2nd. ed. Williams and Wilkins, Baltimore, MD.

Mandell, G. L., G. R. Douglas, and J. E. Bennett. 1990. *Principles and practice of infectious diseases.* 3rd ed. Churchill Livingstone, New York, NY.

McFeters, G. A. (ed.). 1990. *Drinking water microbiology: progress and recent developments.* Springer Verlag, New York, NY.

McGinnis, M. R., R. F. D'Amato, and G. A. Land. 1982. *Pictorial handbook of medically important fungi and aerobic actinomycetes.* Praeger, New York, NY.

The medical letter handbook of antimicrobial therapy. 1990. The Medical Letter, Inc., New Rochelle, NY.

Mims, C. 1987. *The pathogenesis of infectious disease.* 3rd ed. Academic Press, New York, NY.

Morello, J. A., H. E. Mizer, M. E. Wilson, and P. A. Granato. 1994. *Microbiology in patient care.* 5th ed. Wm. C. Brown Communications, Inc., Dubuque, IA.

Noble, E., G. A. Noble, G. A. Schad, and A. J. MacInnes. 1989. *Parasitology: The biology of animal parasites.* 6th ed. Lea & Febiger, Philadelphia, PA.

Perkins, J. J. 1983. *Principles and methods of sterilization in health sciences.* 2nd ed. Charles C Thomas, Springfield, IL.

Rippon, J. W. 1988. *Medical mycology: The pathogenic fungi and the pathogenic actinomycetes.* 3rd ed. W. B. Saunders, Philadelphia, PA.

Rose, N. R., et al. 1992. *Manual of clinical laboratory immunology.* 4th. ed. American Society for Microbiology, Washington, D.C.

Sheehan, C. 1990. *Clinical immunology: principles and laboratory diagnosis.* Lippincott, Philadelphia, PA.

Shulman, S. T., J. P. Phair, and H. M. Sommers. 1992. *The biologic and clinical basis of infectious diseases.* 4th ed. W. B. Saunders, Philadelphia, PA.

Spencer, I. M. and L. S. Monroe. 1982. *The color atlas of intestinal parasites.* 2nd ed. Charles C Thomas, Springfield, IL.

Standard methods for the examination of dairy products. 17th ed. 1989. American Public Health Association, Washington, D.C.

Standard methods for the examination of water and waste water. 17th ed. 1989. American Public Health Association, Washington, D.C.